THE MEDICAL MARIJUANA GUIDE

NATURES PHARMACY

By Chef Derek Butt

Disclaimer

This book is a guide to help you determine the best course of action when it comes to holistic and natural remedies.

I am a licensed medical marijuana producer licensed to grow medical marijuana for medical reasons. The information contained in this book is in no way shape or form intended for illegal use.

This book is a source of information for educational purposes.

The term medical marijuana is a term created by Health Canada in reference to what they identify as legal marijuana.

For serious illnesses you should consult a doctor before using any remedies in this book.

In some countries and in some regions of particular countries, medical marijuana is illegal. I am not advising you to break the law.

Any attempt to utilize medicinal marijuana must be done at your own risk.

I advise you to consult a doctor and acquire the appropriate licensing before using medicinal marijuana.

I am not responsible in any way shape or form, for any loss or legal ramifications incurred by anyone while using medicinal marijuana, or from using the information contained in this book.

Dedication

I wrote this book in honor of my parents who I lost too cancer. I believe the cancer did not kill them, the treatment killed them and I believe if I knew then what I know now, they would still be alive today.

Copyright 2014

Chef Derek Butt.

Table of Contents

Introduction To Medical Marijuana

The use of medical marijuana has been well documented for over eight thousand years. Ancient civilizations have evolved and thrived around the marijuana plant. The marijuana plant has commercial, industrial, medical, nutritional and recreational benefits. All you need is weed.

The Spanish introduced marijuana to South America. Marijuana is Mary Jane in Spanish. The herb moved north up into Mexico along with the knowledge and its medicinal benefits that came with the plant.

When marijuana finally seeped into America it was demonized and became illegal, butt marijuana continued to grow in popularity. At that time, when the U.S. government was busy demonizing marijuana, the public accepted it. They where fooled into thinking that smoking marijuana led to deprivation. Meanwhile, marijuana was commonly known by the American public as cannabis and cannabis extracts was commonly and legally prescribed for many ailments.

Currently, after several decades of research, scientists studying the effects of cannabis made several important discoveries. Not only did they identify the active ingredients in marijuana, they also discovered where and how they work in the brain, via a system called the endocannabinoid system.

The Endocannabinoid System

The endocannabinoid system is a communications network located in the brain and body that affects important functions, including how a person feels, think, and behave.

The natural chemicals produced by the body that interact with the endocannabinoid system are called cannabinoids and like THC and CBD, they interact with receptors to regulate these bodily functions.

Brain cells (neurons) communicate with each other and with the body by sending chemical messages. These messages co-ordinate and regulate everything we feel, think and do. These chemicals (called neurotransmitters) are released from a neuron (a presynaptic cell), move across a small gap (the synapse), and attach to receptors located on a nearby neuron (postsynaptic cell). This triggers a set of events that passes the message along.

The endocannabinoid system communicates in a different way. It receives chemical messages. When the postsynaptic neuron is activated, cannabinoids, (chemical messengers of the enndocannabinoid system) are made on demand from lipid precursors (fat cells) already present in the neuron. They are then released from that cell and travel back and forth to the presynaptic neuron, where they attach to cannabinoid receptors.

Since cannabinoids act on presynaptic cells, they can control what happens next when these cells are activated. In general, cannabinoids function like a regulator for presynaptic neurons, regulating the amount of neurotransmitter (e.g., dopamine) that is released, which affects how messages are sent, received and processed by the cell.

Medicinal marijuana feeds our endocannabinoid system, whether we like it or not, we are all hard wired to thrive on cannabinoids.

The body naturally produces cannabinoids, but with the onslaught of the industrial revolution, the fast food industry, chemical insecticides and pharmaceutical drugs have overwhelmed our immune system. Our bodies can't keep up with the constant exposure of toxins that don't belong in our body.

Fortunately the marijuana plant produces abundant amounts of cannabinoids that our endocannabinoid system thrives on. The brain will begin to communicate and begin to holistically restore physiological balance. The body begins to heal and will prevent as well as cure dis-ease.
There is substantial research by many scientists who can prove that medical marijuana can alleviate many different diseases.

We are learning from these scientists, but when it comes down to it, marijuana does not treat the disease, marijuana treats the body. The body treats the dis-ease, naturally, as nature intended.

Cannabinoids treat our symptoms by identifying the problems and fixing them.

Isolating marijuana compounds and marketing them as medications is not very effective. Like most pharmaceuticals, they have harmful side effects that could result in death.

Marijuana compounds interact and respond to your bodies needs. Isolating compounds is like creating a symphony orchestra with one instrument, or trying to ride a bike with just one wheel.

Marijuana in its natural form is a very powerful medicine with no known harmful side effects.

Marijuana, is not just an effective natural medicine, it is also one of the most nutritious plants in the world. Marijuana is a complete protein with ten amino fatty acids. Marijuana is a "super food."

Neurogenesis

Cannabidiol (CBD), the main non-psychoactive component of the marijuana plant/cannabis, exerts therapeutically promising effects on human mental health such as inhibition of psychosis, anxiety and depression.

Cannabinoids promote embryonic and adult hippocampus neurogenesis and produce anxiolytic and antidepressant like effects.

The hippocampal dentate gyrus in the adult mammalian brain contains neural stem/progenitor cells, capable of generating new neurons, i.e., neurogenesis. These newborn hippocampal neurons are functionally integrated into the existing neuroanatomical circuitry and are positively correlated with hippocampus-dependent learning and memory processes and the developmental mechanisms of stress and mood disorders.

Most drugs examined to date like opiates, alcohol, nicotine and cocaine decrease adult hippocampal neurogenesis but the effects of marijuana on hippocampal neurogenesis is positive.

With the aid of cannabis and the endocannabinoid system the hippocampus can produce thousands of new cells a day throughout your adult life.

Marijuana regulates neurogenesis. The cannabinoids found in marijuana appear to be the only medicinal compound with the capacity to produce increased hippocampal newborn neurons. Grow a brain or go insane. Just kidding. Laughter is good medicine.

Marijuana doesn't cause brain damage, marijuana repairs brain damage.

Marijuana is a neuro protector and is positively correlated with its anxiolytic and antidepressant effects.

Regeneration

The body has the ability to regenerate. That means the body is capable of healing itself if it has the right elements to function. These elements come from the food you eat, the water you drink, the air you breathe, the light you see and the energy you feel. When the body has all the elements that it needs to function, the mind and body regenerates as sure as a cut heals on your skin.

The new science and the new medical model will focus on restoring physiological balance so the body can heal itself rather then just administer toxic drugs that will most likely make the condition worse. A treated disease has up to four times the fatality rate then an untreated disease. It would be unfair to say that any disease is left untreated because breathing, eating, drinking or any environmental stimulus is some form of treatment.

Disease is caused by three things. Toxicity, a deficiency and or nerve damage. The nervous system regulates every system in the body. The nervous system is referred to by doctors as the Neurological system. Toxic means poison so Neurotoxicity are poisoned nerves from a toxic condition. So the first step is to cleanse the system, clean the blood, flush those toxins out, the way you would flush your plants out to maintain healthy vigorous growth. The next step is to nourish the body with the nutrients that it needs to grow and restore physiological balance.

Marijuana is a complete food source and an anti oxidant. Fresh raw marijuana consumed as a source of food will restore balance, the body will regenerate itself back to a healthy state. In essence marijuana has the potential to heal 97% of all diseases because marijuana provides you with the elements that your body needs to heal itself.

Genetic diseases are very rare, less then 3% so most diseases are preventable, reversible and curable. It doesn't matter what disease you have because with the new medical model and the new science, all diseases are treated the same way. Detox and nourish the system. Rest and rejuvenation. Exercise mind and body. It's all about rebuilding your physiology from the inside out.

It also doesn't matter what strain of marijuana you use, every strain is different but they are all basically the same. From a scientists perspective any marijuana plant will heal you.

With all of this said, the body doesn't say I have cancer and I need chemotherapy, It sais I am toxic and I need to be cleansed and nourished.

Top Ten Health Benefits

1. CANCER
Cannabinoids inhibit tumor growth and kill cancer cells. Our governments have known this for some time and they continue to suppress the information.

2.TOURRETTE'S SYNDROME
Tourette's syndrome is a neurological condition characterized by uncontrollable body movements. Dr. Kirsten Mueller-Vahl of the Hanover Medical College in Germany investigated the effects of cannabinols in 12 adult Tourette's patients. A single dose of the cannabinol produced a reduction in symptoms for several hours.

3. SEIZURES
Fresh Raw Marijuana is a muscle relaxant with "antispasmodic" qualities that have proven to be an effective treatment for seizures. There are countless cases of people suffering from seizures that have been able to function better through the use of fresh raw marijuana.

4. MIGRAINES
Since the legalization of medicinal marijuana California doctors have been able to treat more than 300,000 cases of migraines without the use of conventional medicine. I do not get migraine headaches when I eat fresh raw marijuana

5. GLAUCOMA
Medicinal marijuana's treatment of glaucoma has been well documented. There isn't a single valid study that disproves marijuana's powerful effects on glaucoma patients.

6. MULTIPLE SCLEROSIS
Former talk-show host, Montel Williams began to use medicinal marijuana to treat his MS. Medicinal marijuana inhibits the neurological effects and muscle spasms, symptoms of the fatal disease.

7. ADD and ADHD
Medical marijuana is a perfect alternative for Ritalin and treats the disorder without any negative side effects.

8. IBS and CROHNS
Marijuana has shown that it can help with symptoms as it stops nausea, abdominal pain, and diarrhea.

9. ALZHEIMER'S
The Scripps Institute, in 2006, proved that THC found in marijuana works to prevent Alzheimer's by blocking the deposits in the brain that cause the disease.

10.PREMENSTRUAL SYNDROME

Medical marijuana is used to treat cramps and discomfort that causes PMS symptoms. Using marijuana for PMS goes back to the day of Queen Victoria.

Mounting Evidence Suggests Raw Cannabis is Best.

Cannabinoids found in marijuana can prevent cancer and reduce heart attacks by 66% and insulin dependent diabetes by 58%. Cannabis clinician Dr. William Courtney recommends drinking 4 - 8 ounces of raw bud and leaf juice from any hemp or marijuana plant. 5-10 mg of Cannabidiol (CBD) per kg of body weight is recommended by the FDA.

Why raw?

Heat destroys enzymes and nutrients in plants. Fresh raw marijuana allows for a greater availability of these elements. Those who need large amounts of cannabinoids without the psychoactive effect can utilize the medication at 60 times more tolerance than if it were heated.

Raw cannabis is considered to be by experts, a dietary essential. A powerful anti-inflammatory and antioxidant, raw cannabis is a super food, a power food, food that is functional, food that heals. NATURES PHARMACY.

Good health begins in the gut.

Chronic Pain Management

The American of Family Physicians, the American Public Health Association, the American Nurses Association and even the New England Journal of Medicine endorses the use of medical marijuana for the treatment of severe chronic pain. Marijuana is a safe non-addictive anti-inflammatory. Side effects may include the munchies.

Pain relief is what marijuana is most commonly used for. Smoking or vaping cannabis will provide instant relief by up to 30%. If you ingest marijuana you increase its effectiveness by ten fold.

For pain relief you are looking for a strong Indica strain with high levels of THC but it is not THC alone that alleviates pain. Other compounds found in marijuana create a synergy to complete its effects on your physiology. Marijuana will help you relax and help you sleep, which will also reduce inflammation. Cannabis has analgesic properties that make marijuana an effective medicine for chronic pain syndrome.

The problem is doctors do not know how to treat chronic pain. Pain is your friend. Pain is a symptom of an underlying condition, a defense mechanism that lets you know something is wrong. Treating your symptoms with toxic pain killers only makes your condition worse, which is why you have to constantly increase your dosage. An inflammatory state is a toxic condition that needs to be cleaned up with a cleansing diet that will detox and nourish your physiological systems.

I believe *fresh raw marijuana* is more effective as an anti-inflammatory. I am no stranger to pain, after a serious car accident I was left in excruciating pain for several years. Pain killers where not cutting it and using them for extended periods of time is very harmful, so I threw my pain killers in the garbage and bought me some ganga. Finally, I was able to think again.
I recently discovered how powerful fresh raw marijuana is as an anti-inflammatory. Fresh raw marijuana has completely alleviated my migraine headaches and I am able to medicate without getting high. I like the euphoric effects of cannabis but I do not like being high all the time.

I am sixty years old and I am completely pain free. No aches and pains, no arthritis, no migraine headaches and no painkillers. Smoking marijuana will provide you with some relief but for effective pain management you have to start eating and or juicing fresh raw marijuana.

Cannabis root contains very high levels of CBD and is very effective as an anti-inflammatory. Two teaspoons of cannabis root in a smoothie will melt your pain away leaving you feeling relaxed without a heavy THC buzz. You will feel perfectly medicated for most of the day, feeling energetic, happy and feeling good for daytime activities.

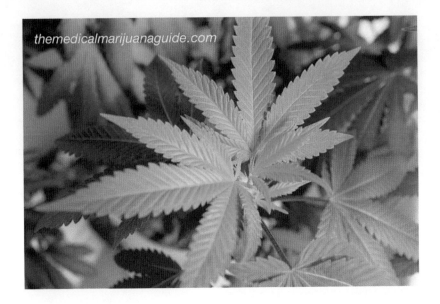

Fresh Raw Marijuana

The first step to recovery is to put your self on a healthy diet. Consuming fresh raw marijuana is probably one of the best things you can do for your mind and body.

Marijuana holistically restores physiological balance, which enables the body to heal itself, which is why it is so effective for many different diseases.

In raw form, marijuana leaves and buds are loaded with a non-psychoactive antioxidant, anti-inflammatory and anti-cancer nutrient compound known as cannabidiol (CBD), that is proving to be a "super food," capable of preventing and reversing chronic illnesses. Large amounts of CBD can also be found in hemp oil.

Marijuana is technically a vegetable, with many medicinal substances and with immune-regulating capabilities. The human body already contains a built-in endogenous cannabinoid system complete with cannabinoid receptors. Ingesting CBD rich marijuana can help restore balance and normalize the body's functional systems, including cell communication and proper immune function.

Fresh raw marijuana is alkaline forming and oxygenates the blood. Disease thrives in an acidic environment so correcting ph balance thru diet will help reverse the disease. It is an important step to recovery.

When you eat or juice fresh raw marijuana you consume close to one hundred percent of its cannabinoid content. THC in its raw form is THCa. Its carbon molecule is still attached and is non-psychoactive. It will not get you high, so you can medicate without any narcotic effects.

The problem with drying, curing and then smoking cannabis is that you loose approximately eighty percent of its cannabinoid content in the process, rendering it less effective as a medication. If you also consider that we are only able to absorb twenty percent of those cannabinoids into our blood stream orally, it becomes even less effective.

According to Dr. Courtney, you should not eat more then eight leaves a day. I will chop up marijuana and eat them with salads but be careful because an acidic dressing could decarboxylate the marijuana, making it psychoactive.

I juice Marijuana or make smoothies. I love smoothies, they are very healthy, nutritious and delicious. I will also add hemp protein powder made from marijuana hemp seeds.

I have experimented with fresh raw marijuana, tinctures and cannabis oil. I have found consuming marijuana fresh and raw to be very effective as a medicine and vital for recovery. I have also recently discovered that cannabis paste is also very effective.

I have also discovered that cannabinoids heal the mind, as well as the body, since most cannabinoid receptors are located in the brain. I have experienced a remarkable improvement in my cognitive abilities, plus I am more stable emotionally. I can think clearly and I am starting to see the bigger picture.

I have published a few videos online on eating and juicing fresh raw marijuana.

You can view them on my YouTube channel, Chef Derek Butt or you can view them on my website at chefderekbutt.com or themedicalmarijuanaguide.com

Fresh Raw Marijuana Nutrition

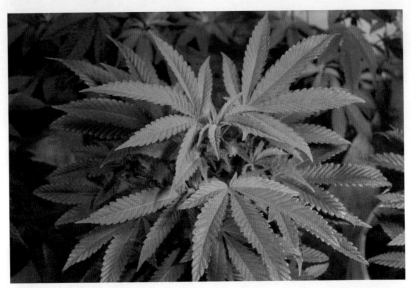

Fresh raw marijuana is a complete food source. No other single plant source has the essential amino acids in such an easily digestible form, providing instant food energy. Fresh raw marijuana contains all the essential amino acids and fatty acids necessary in maintaining life. Fresh raw marijuana has the perfect 3-1 ratio of omega 6 and 3 fatty acids.

Fresh raw marijuana is an abundant supply of nutrients like magnesium, Phytosterols, Ascorbic Acid, Beta Carotene, Calcium, Folic Acid, Fiber, Iron, Potassium, Phosphorus, Zinc, Riboflavin, Niacin and Thiamine.

Fresh raw marijuana is also rich in vitamin A, E, D and B12.

The Amino Acids in fresh raw marijuana is a good source of digestible protein.

Fresh raw marijuana is beneficial for skin conditions like sunburn, acme, eczema and psoriasis. Fresh raw marijuana rejuvenates the skin. Fresh raw marijuana relieves symptoms of PMS and is an effective anti-inflammatory that provides pain relieve.

Fresh raw marijuana provides instant energy and reduces fatigue.

Fresh raw marijuana improves memory, concentration and alertness.

Fresh raw marijuana improves emotional stability and cognitive abilities. Fresh raw marijuana increases your learning abilities.

Fresh raw marijuana will prevent disease and balance your immune system.

The big question is, where do I get my hands on fresh raw marijuana? Well you pretty much have to grow your own, if it can be done legally. Grow your herb organically under full spectrum light for best results. Natural sunlight produces the best medicine. Check out my book The Medical Marijuana Growers Guide and start producing your own medicine. Take healthcare into your own hands. Some growers grow organically in a healthy growing environment but not all growers grow for the same reasons. if growing your own is not an option, find a grower that can provide you with the quality you are looking for.

I have published a few videos online on eating and juicing fresh raw marijuana. Here is a link to my fresh raw marijuana Video. Eating Fresh Raw Marijuana

Marijuana Salads

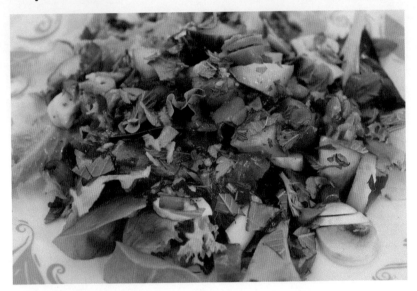

Salads should be a large part of our diet. Go for the dark leafy greens and that includes fresh raw marijuana. Don't be afraid to add fresh vegetables, fruits, nuts, seeds, legumes and sprouts. Get creative with it. You could even slice up some animal based protein and add that to your salad. Variety is key.

Oil and Vinegar Dressing

Crush a clove of fresh garlic, dice up a few green olives and add it to a bowl. Add about 3 tbsp. of olive oil, 2 tbsp. of vinegar and about 3 tbsp. of fresh lemon juice. Mix in the bowl. Season to taste with sea salt and black pepper. Add about a 1/4 tsp. of crushed chilies to heat it up a little. The lemon juice may decarboxylate the fresh raw marijuana in your salad. You could also add a pinch of basil and or oregano or perhaps some fresh mint. To make this dressing psychoactive just replace some of the olive oil with cannabis infused olive oil. This recipe will make one or two servings.

Basic French Mayonnaise

I am going to show you how to make a basic French mayonnaise because it is the foundation for most salad dressings.

Before we begin, whenever we are working with raw eggs in our recipe you have to pasteurize the eggs first. If you don't, you have a 20% chance of getting infected with salmonella and it could be fatal for some. To prevent infection, heat up a pan of water and place the eggs in the water for approximately ten minutes at 180ºF. This will kill most of the bacteria and reduce the risk of infection. It is important that the internal temperature of the egg reaches 180ºF for ten minutes.

For best results, I start with clean cold utensils. I place my bowl and whisk in the fridge before hand.

Add a quarter teaspoon of dry mustard in a cold bowl. Add one pasteurized egg and start whisking vigorously while slowly pouring in one cup of light tasting olive oil. The oil will emulsify and get thicker, at this point add one or two tablespoons of unpasteurized apple cider vinegar to thin out the dressing a little. Add a clove of fresh crushed garlic, a tablespoon of fresh lemon juice and season to taste with sea salt and black pepper. Some chefs will use white pepper but I just don't like white pepper.

So there you have it, basic French mayonnaise. I have tried substituting some or all of the olive oil with cannabis infused olive oil and the mayonnaise broke.

You can chop up fresh herbs like fresh raw marijuana, basil, parsley or whatever and add that to the mix. You could add Parmesan cheese and capers and make it a Caesar dressing. You could add a couple of tablespoons of tomato paste for a French dressing, some tomato paste and relish for a Thousand-Island dressing. You could add blue cheese for a Blue Cheese dressing. Get creative with it.

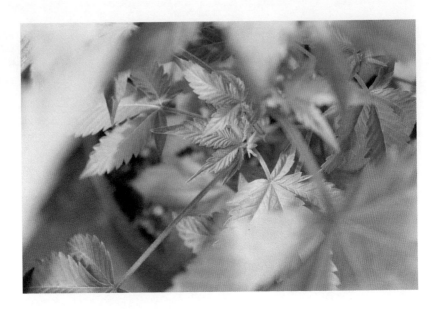

Juicing Fresh Raw Marijuana

Juicing marijuana is traditionally done in a juicer. Personally I find the method to be slow, plus they extract the fiber from the plant, which contains nutrition, minerals and medicinal compounds. However, the end product is very potent and rich in chlorophyll for oxygenation.

Mix an ounce of marijuana juice with eight ounces of vegetable and or fruit juice, or juice the marijuana with other fruits and vegetables.

This juice will not get you high. Marijuana in its natural form is non-psychoactive and does not become a narcotic until it begins to decarboxylate.

Be careful not to allow the juice to heat up. Marijuana begins to decarboxylate at 175° F and if it does, eight ounces of marijuana juice would be equivalent to a thousand joints according to Dr. Courtney, a leading scientist in medical marijuana research.

I juice marijuana in a high-speed 1400 w. blender. Some people claim that the high speed generates enough heat to decarboxylate the marijuana and break down enzymes but these people probably lack the experience of using a high-speed blender. I throw in a few ice cubes to prevent this from happening. The blender is so fast the marijuana is juiced in a few short pulses. I prefer this method because you retain fiber in the juice and you could strain it off, if you where so inclined to do so.

Check out my YouTube channel or my website for a video on "Juicing Fresh Raw Marijuana". Here is the link.

Juicing Fresh Raw Marijuana

Marijuana Smoothies

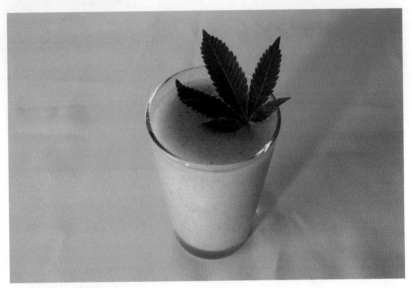

Marijuana Smoothies is how I do most of my medicating. Even though I have made some green vegetable smoothies and fruit and vegetable smoothies, I prefer fruit smoothies.

I have made a remarkable recovery, in mind and body by drinking a smoothie, once a day. I have more energy, I am more alert, I am more stable emotionally, my memory has improved and my skin condition has improved. I had cysts that have cleared up and I do not get any more migraine headaches. It feels good to be alive again.

For a single portion, I start out adding a few ice cubes into the blender then I will add my fruit. Now I will add three to five Marijuana leaves. Dr. Courtney recommends you don't eat more then eight leaves a day. For a boost I will add a teaspoon of hemp protein powder made from hemp seed. I may add some honey for its nutritional and medicinal benefits but it is not necessary as a sweetener.

Ok, now we need a few ounces of liquid. What you choose is up to you, you could use coconut milk, hemp milk, and or almond milk. There is much to choose from. I use hemp milk. Just don't use cows milk unless it is unpasteurized and raw, meaning unprocessed. The best way to drink cows milk is to just suck on the cow's tit. We are the only species who drinks breast milk from another species and we are the only species who drinks breast milk in adulthood so it might look a little odd.

Now that we have our liquid of choice in hand, pour a few ounces in the blender and pulse a few times. Your smoothie should be ready for consumption.

To view a video on how to make smoothies please visit my YouTube channel.

Marijuana Smoothie with Hemp Milk

The Marijuana Mango with cows milk.

Cannabis

Cannabis is the cured dried flower of the marijuana plant, commonly known as bud. Most people will smoke or vaporize the bud for a euphoric effect but most of its medicinal properties deteriorate in the process.

A more efficient way to medicate is to ingest cannabis by making natural remedies like cannabis oil, hash, tinctures, canna oil, cannabis paste and cannabis butter. From these extracts and infusions you can make an endless list of marijuana edibles.

People smoke or vaporize cannabis. Both methods of smoking cannabis is just as effective medicinally, with vaporizing there is less carcinogens to deal with. You can also control the temperature of the burn and target certain cannabinoids with a vaporizer. Know your numbers.

Regardless of smoking and vaporizing inefficiencies and efficiencies, smoking or vaporizing cannabis has many health benefits. Smoking cannabis is very therapeutic, even when smoked recreationally.
Marijuana does not stop becoming a medication when consumed for recreational reasons.

Smoking or vaporizing cannabis will not correct the imbalance that caused your symptoms to begin with but smoking cannabis provides instant relieve and the dosage is controllable. Smoking or vaporizing provides instant relieve for a wide array of symptoms.

There are many hybrid strains of Cannabis to choose from and they are basically Indica, or Sativa crosses. Pure Indicas are sedative and numbing, while pure Sativas are uplifting and creative.

For medicinal purposes, you are looking for a strain that is rich in CBD. a non-psychoactive ingredient with powerful health benefits.
Some strains like Charlottes Web or Cannatonic contain higher levels of CBD, which are highly sought after for serious illnesses. CBD is a regulator and will identify THC as a toxin and balance out its narcotic effect on the body.

CBD Rich Strains

Critical Mass. 5% CBD
CBD Skunk Haze. 5% CBD
Nordle. 5.5% CBD
Shark. 6% CBD
Charlottes web. 17-23% CBD
Cannatonic. 25% CBD

These numbers are estimates. The numbers will change from grower to grower, which depends on the environment and how they where bred and raised. Most or all CBD rich strains are Cannatonic strains developed in Amsterdam.

Drying And Curing

After you remove the foliage from the plant, hang the bud on its stem, upside down, in a dark, well-ventilated room, with moderate humidity. Dry the plants for up to two weeks. The slower the better and after cutting and manicuring, cure your bud in a glass jar or a brown paper bag for up to a couple of months or more, the slower the better. You will have to open the jars for a few minutes, up to a few times a day, depending on the moisture content of the Cannabis. This is like a fermentation process and starches convert into sugars. Drying and curing marijuana is an art unto itself and I go into it in more detail in my Medical Marijuana Growers guide.

Once the cannabis is prepared properly you will be able to enjoy a sweet tasting smoke.

Decarboxylation

When Marijuana dries and cures, it still is not a narcotic. It is non-psychoactive until you decarboxylate it. At this point THCa still has its carbon molecule attached. THCa doesn't decarboxylate until you light it up, burn it, or cook or extract it with heat. Cannabis, the cured dried flower of the marijuana plant technically is not a narcotic.

Cannabis begins to decarboxylate at 175° F and begins to deteriorate at 220° F. Cannabis does not become a narcotic until you apply heat.

If you eat cannabis without cooking it first, you should not
get high but the acids in your stomach may decarboxylate the cannabis to some degree. Also if the grower placed their lights too close too the plants while growing, the heat from the lights could decarboxylate the herb.

Decarboxylation is a process that uses heat to release the acid molecule, turning THCa into THC.

To decarboxylate or not is the question. I recommend not to decarboxylate for most medical reasons, however sometimes a narcotic effect is necessary. I talk about decarboxilation in this video. Check it out. Cannabutter revised

Smoking Cannabis For The First Time

Smoking cannabis for the first time could be nerve wrecking if you have been misinformed. When you smoke cannabis for the first time you will probably not get high. That is how it worked for myself and others I knew at the time.

When you do get high for the first time, you will laugh your head off uncontrollably. You will have a great time, the time of your life. All that laughter is like purging your system of a lifetime of stress.

Once you build up a resistance, this doesn't happen anymore and this is where some people can get emotionally, or psychologically attached but cannabis is not biologically addictive.

The first high is the best high, you will never get that back and some of you could end up spending the rest of your lives trying to re-live that experience and it is never going to happen so except that and move on.

Once you build up a resistance, you can enjoy marijuana for what it is. No more uncontrollable laughter, just a deep relaxed feeling of wellbeing. Once you go thru this process, you realize that cannabis is not a hard drug like alcohol, which places people out of control.

Alcohol is a narcotic. Eighty percent of all crime is committed under the influence of alcohol. Alcohol is responsible for so much domestic violence. We are a drug ridden society and the one thing that can alleviate some of these problems is illegal and for no good reason.

"When we end the prohibition on marijuana we can begin fighting the war on drugs."

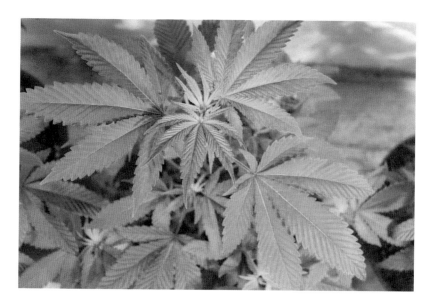

Indica or Sativa

The effects of smoking Cannabis is euphoric, sedative and can vary from strain to strain. There are many strains out there and for medicinal applications you need a strain that is rich in CBD. CBD is a regulator and will reduce THC content.

There are two basic strains that are commonly used and there are many hybrids of the two strains. There is a third strain Ruderallis, it is adapted for winter climates but the THC content is very low.

The most common of the two strains is Indica. Indica strains have broad leafs and are short, fat and bushy with a short growth cycle. Indoor growers prefer growing Indica or a strong Indica / Sativa hybrid.

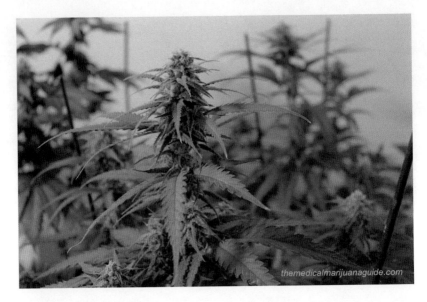

themedicalmarijuanaguide.com

Sativa has thin leaf blades, which has a longer growth cycle and grows up to twenty-five feet in a season. Indoor growers will avoid growing Sativa but there are hybrids that have adapted for indoor growing. A pure Sativa strain is rare.

Each strain has its own range of effects on the mind and body, resulting in a wide range of medicinal benefits.

The effect produced from smoking Indica bud is a strong physical body effect that will make you sleepy and provides a deep relaxed feeling, compared to the Sativa effect, which is known to be more energetic and uplifting. Because Sativa and Indica strains have very different medicinal benefits and effects, certain strains can be targeted to better treat specific illnesses.

Indica dominant marijuana strains tend to have a strong sweet, or sour aroma to the buds (ex. Kush, OG Kush) providing a very relaxing and strong body high that is helpful in treating general anxiety, body pain, eating and sleeping disorders.

Medical marijuana patients smoke Indica in the late evening, or right before bed due to how sleepy and tired you become when high from an Indica strain like Kush.

Benefits of Cannabis Indica

1. Relieves body pain 2. Relaxes muscles 3. Relieves spasms, reduces seizures 4. Relieves headaches and migraines 5. Relieves anxiety or stress

Sativa dominant marijuana strains tend to have a more grassy type odor to the buds, providing an uplifting, energetic and cerebral effect that is best suited for daytime smoking. A sativa high is one filled with creativity. Many artists take advantage of the creative powers of Cannabis Sativa.

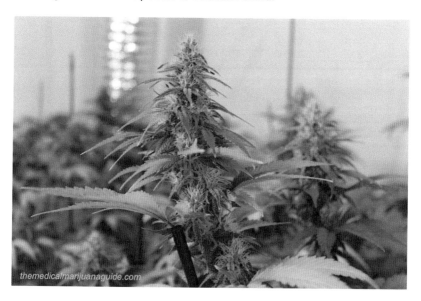

Benefits of Cannabis Sativa

1. Feelings of well being and at-ease
2. Uplifting and cerebral
3. Stimulates and energizes
4. Increases focus and creativity
5. Alleviates depression.

Cannabis stimulates your appetite so if you are obese you can curve those food cravings with a glass of water. If you have many snacks during the day instead of three large meals you could actually eat more and loose weight.

If you are anorexic you won't be for long.

Over all, cannabis has many health benefits and I find it therapeutic even if just smoked for recreational reasons. I find that smoking smaller amounts (less more often) leaves me more energetic and alert.

Legalizing Marijuana

Legalizing marijuana will change the world. It will fuel are economy, while helping us live a better, healthier, more productive and sustainable life style. We will become less dependent on oil and other depleted resources and more independent.

There is a major shift in power going on in our society today. Governments have to start thinking what is best for people and not cold hearted corporations with no soul.

We are at a pinnacle in our society. Do we take the high road and build a healthy sustainable economy or do we take the low road and let corporations drain are wealth and drive us into the ground.

We have to educate our governments before corporations completely take over. We have to bring them out of the dark ages and into the new world, a new age of enlightenment.

84% of our economy is built on the backbone of the small independent businessperson. The mom and pop operation so if you look at the big picture, corporations do not add up to much. There power is an illusion.

The Marijuana industry is bigger then all other industries put together so the world elite are really small players in the big picture. Again, their power is an illusion.

The Marijuana industry is a horizontal collective unlike our society, which is a hierarchy, a vertical collective adopted by most animal species with the exception of the Canadian Beaver. A horizontal collective is not centralized, everybody has equal opportunity and everybody works cooperatively for the common good of all, much like a family. However, in a vertical collective, people are forced to compete as individuals for power and social acceptability.

If the federal government de-scheduled marijuana, society as we know it will crumble. People will have the power to live independently from the shackles of society and a new world will immerge. A world of peace, harmony and prosperity for all.

As a species we claim to be different from animals but that difference is not by much. Our DNA is 98% chimpanzee. That 2% is two chromosomes that have been bonded together. This does not happen naturally in nature. We have been genetically modified and I can assure you it was not done by our species. My question is, who owns the patent?

Ok, back to reality.

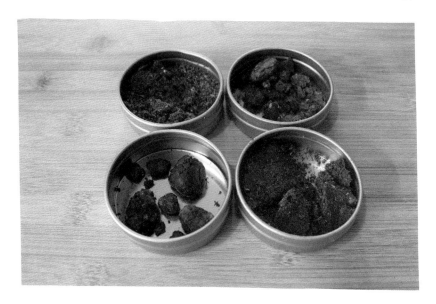

Hashish

Hash is the resin from the plant. The marijuana plant is covered in resin and is mostly concentrated in the bud. There are many ways to make hash but I will cover the most popular methods.

Chalice

Chalice is what you see in the above picture. It is hash made from the resin of the live plant. Usually it is collected from your fingers or gloves by rubbing them together. I guess this would be the safest and most pure form of extraction there is. It happens naturally when you handle the plant but some farmers will rub their plants with their hands to extract the resin and then rub their hands together to make chalice. I should do a video on this.

Bubble Hash

Making bubble hash takes a fair amount of time and work and you do loose some of the terpenes in the water.

Bubble hash is made from a cold-water extraction process, which preserves cannabinoids. I prefer using hash over hash oil if heat or solvent was used in the extraction process.

To make bubble hash you will need a container with lots of ice and cold water. You will need a set of bubble bags. Start with the largest size bag, which is 220 microns. Place the bag in the container with enough ice and some water to make a slurry. Place fresh frozen or dried frozen marijuana in the container of ice and cold water. Stir with a beater for three or four minutes. Some people will rig up an electric drill with an attachment that stirs stucco.
The mix should be a golden brown color. Stop mixing before the mix turns green, about three or four minutes. By this time most of the ice should be melted and you are ready to pour the mix thru your filtration bags.

You could do a second pass with fresh water and ice to increase your yield.

The filtration bags are called bubble bags and they come in different sizes. You usually get several filtration bags in a kit ranging in mesh sizes from 220 microns down to 20 microns.

Place you bags in a clean container starting with the smallest filter first and work down to the largest filter in the inside. Pour your mix into the bags. It could take up to an hour for the mix to filter thru.

Once done you are ready to remove the hash.

Use rubber gloves when handling the hash and place the hash on a sheet of paper to dry out. Once dry, it can be packed and stored.

Hash retrieved from the larger bags are used for infusing into food and the finer grade hash retrieved from 190 microns down to 20 microns are used for infusing into beverages.

Even though I have showed you how to make cannabis oil using heat and solvents, I believe that hash made thru a cold-water extraction to be a far superior product medicinally. Bubble hash is cleaner and more potent.

Dry Sift Hash

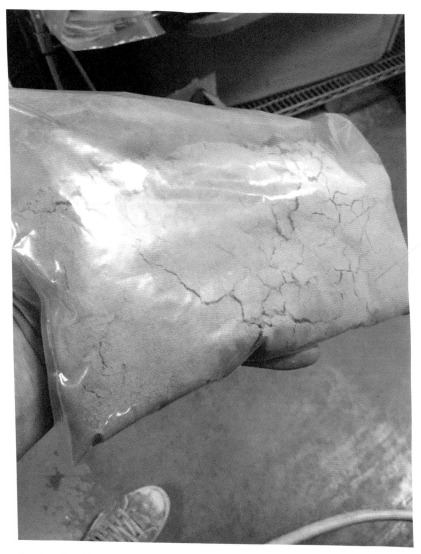

Making dry sift hash is easier to make and you do not loose any terpenes in the water. You will need a screen mounted on a wooden frame. A 120 micron screen will work but some people will use a 90 micron screen for better quality. Freeze your dried marijuana 24 hours in advance and place the marijuana on the screen. This should be done on glass so you can scrape the kief off the glass.

Shimmy the filter and move around the marijuana so the trichomes will fall of the plant and thru the screen. This could take thirty minutes to an hour. Once you have rendered the kief, scrape it up and compress it into hash. Use rubber gloves when handling the hash to prevent it from going moldy in storage. In a few days, the hash will get darker in color from oxidization.

The idea is to make your extracts as potent as possible. This way you will only need small amounts to meet your dosage requirements without affecting too much of the taste of the food or beverages that you are preparing.

Shatter

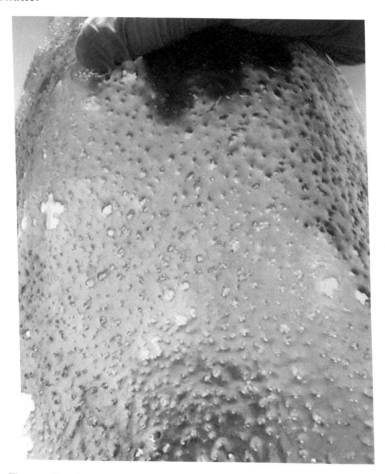

The quality of shatter has improved greatly since butane is now sold in food grade cans. Shatter is basically a butane extraction. The extraction must be done outside. Butane is very volatile, so wear a mask. You don't want to breathe in those vapors. The extraction tube gets freezing cold so wear protective gloves.

Freeze your herb and pack your extraction tube fairly snug but not to snug. Strap on a filter (most people will use a coffee filter) at the open end of the tube.

Turn on your heat pad and fan before you start playing with butane. Any kind of static charge or spark could enlighten you but not in a good way.

Inject the butane thru the small hole at the other end of the tube. Allow butane to flow evenly down the tube into a Pyrex dish. The liquid should come out a golden brown color. Some people will do a second pass.

Evaporate the alcohol. Most people will use a water bath at about 90-110°F. This also should be done outside. You can use a heat pad on a medium setting. As the butane evaporates, the resin will form bubbles and you are left with cannabis resin that is a clear golden color. If you want to make shatter, cook at lower temps, if you want to make honeycomb, cook at slightly higher temps. Make sure you are consistent with the heat. You can let the resin sit for twenty-four hours to purge the butane. Some people will then whip it up to make budda. If moisture gets into the mix, your extract will turn opaque.

If you want to make shatter don't mess with it. The resin is still a tar like consistency and can be scraped off with a fresh razor blade. Spread a thin layer of the cannabis resin onto parchment paper.

Place the parchment paper with the cannabis resin in a vacuum chamber with a consistent heat supply or better yet, a vacuum oven. Cook the cannabis for about six hours at about 90°F. The resin will initially bubble up and form a muffin shape. It is very important to achieve this on the first purge.

At this point, it can be whipped into budda or you can purge for another six hours until your cannabis extract turns into shatter.

At this point you should be able to handle it without it sticking to your fingers and it should shatter when you drop it on a counter top.

When you handle the product, it would be a good idea to wear latex gloves, use sterile tools and work on a frozen slab of marble.

When smoking shatter, it is a good idea to have a glass bong and a butane torch so you can achieve a full melt.

The quality of your shatter depends allot on the herb you use. OG Kush is a good strain to use for shatter. If you use buds for starting material, obviously the finished product will be better and more yielding then if you used shake.

I just gave you the basic guide. The timing, the temperatures, the consistency of the temperatures and how you handle the product will determine how the product turns out. Making shatter is an art unto itself. With practice you will be able to master it.

Cannabis Oil

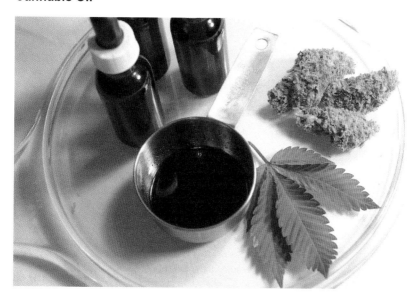

Cannabis oil has been around for thousands of years but Rick Simpson has recently brought it into the public eye. As (RSO) Rick Simpson Oil. He discovered that it cures cancer.

Scientists have known about cannabis oil for some time now. Doctors frequently prescribed cannabis before it became illegal back in the late forties, early fifties. At that time the general public new marijuana as cannabis as it was in many house hold products and medications.

Laboratory tests conducted in 2008 by a team of scientists showed that the active ingredient in marijuana, known as tetrahydrocannabinol or THC can cure brain cancer by inducing human glioma cell death through autophagy. The study concluded that the same biochemical process, THC could alleviate multiple types of cancers, affecting various cells in the body. Other studies have shown that cannabinoids terminates cell growth, inducing cell death, and inhibiting tumor metastasis. What is amazing is that while cannabinoids effectively target and kill cancerous cells, they do not affect healthy cells and may actually protect them against cellular death. Moreover, cannabinoids are also researched for their anti-inflammatory abilities as they bind to receptors in the brain, much like opioid derivatives that are commonly prescribed today.

Further evidence to support the effects of cannabis extract on malignant cells comes from the many real life experiences of individuals, who have successfully overcome cancer by using cannabis oil.

Examples include a patient, who managed to completely cure his skin cancer by simply applying cannabis oil onto the affected areas of the skin, as well as another, who recovered from a severe head injury with the aid of hemp oil.

One of the cannabinoids that has displayed amazing medical properties is cannabidiol, or CBD a non-psychoactive compound that is regarded by some as the medical discovery of the 21st century and with good reason. Research indicates that CBD can relieve convulsions, reduce inflammation, lower anxiety and suppress nausea, while also inhibiting cancer development. In addition, CBD has exhibited neuroprotective properties, relieving symptoms of dystonia and proving just as effective as regular antipsychotics in the treatment of schizophrenia and other mental illnesses, like bi-polar disorder. CBD alone is very ineffective without the synergy that is created from other compounds found in marijuana like THC. The whole plant must be used for effective results.

What stands out is that from the vast amount of research and data available, as well as the personal experiences of cancer survivors, is that no chemotherapy currently being used medically can match the non-toxic, anti-carcinogenic and anti-tumorigenic effects of these natural plant compounds.

Cannabis oil is a concentrated form of the marijuana plant and is not to be confused with hemp oil, or Canna Oil. Cannabis oil has a much higher cannabinoid content, rendering it more effective as a medicine.

You can smoke cannabis oil but it is primarily consumed and ingested orally as a medicine. The most efficient way to medicate with cannabis oil is to ingest the oil, raw. Undecarboxylated.

Cannabis Oil Dosage Information

For most adults, you will need 60 grams of cannabis oil to kill the cancer. For the average person, it will take about 90 days to ingest the full 60-gram treatment of cannabis oil. Start small with three doses of cannabis oil per day. Each dose should be the size of a half a grain of rice. After one week you should be able to double the dose you are taking. The dose should be doubled every four days, until 1 gram per day can be ingested.

This way of dosing the oil allows the body to build up a tolerance. You can slightly reduce your dosage during the day hours and slightly increase your dosage before bed. This will help in gaining quality of sleep. We all have different tolerances for any medication.

The size and body weight of a person has little to do with your tolerance to cannabis oil, but does affect the amount of dosage that should be used.

Be aware that when treating with cannabis oil, it is also likely it will lower your blood pressure. If you are currently taking blood pressure medication, it's possible you will no longer need to take it. Once you start the cannabis oil, make sure to monitor your blood pressure.

At the end of treatment, continued use of the cannabis oil for awhile is a good idea. At that time it should be at a reduced dosage. Taking one gram per month is a good dose to maintain your health.

The main side effect most people experience with cannabis oil is sleep and rest. Both play important roles in healing mind and body. Within an hour of taking a dose of cannabis oil, the oil will cause people to get tired. Don't fight it, just use that time to rest.
Usually within the first 30 days the daytime sleepiness that is experienced reduces as you build a resistance but the patient continues to sleep very well during the night.

Starting with larger doses could be good to help patients get off addictive and dangerous pain medications, like Morphine or Vicodin. When people, using those types of medications start the cannabis oil treatment, they could cut their pain medications by as much as half. It might also be good to start with larger doses if the cancer is in the late stages.

Most importantly though you always want to make sure you stay within your comfort zone when taking the cannabis oil. Everyone is different, some people can take more than others. Make sure the dose you take is right for you.

Cannabis oil has a very high success rate in the treatment of cancer. Unfortunately, many people who decide to start cannabis oil treatment have been badly damaged by chemo and radiation. That damage done by those treatments can extend the time and the amount of cannabis oil needed to kill cancer. Depending on the damage done and type of cancer, it could take as much as 180 grams of cannabis oil to kill the cancer.

The oil is also able to rejuvenate vital organs in the body, like the pancreas. Some diabetics who have taken the oil find that after about six weeks of treating with cannabis oil that they have reduced their insulin use in half. In certain cases, they no longer require insulin at all, since their pancreas started functioning.

Cannabis is very complex and how you metabolize these compounds is unique to you. The dosage information is meant to be a guide. It is up to you to take health care into your hands and decide what dosage works best for you. Start small and increase your dosage slowly.

Treating Skin Cancer

You will need about an ounce of high quality cannabis to make the oil to treat skin cancer. With this amount of starting material you should get 3 to 4 grams of high-grade cannabis oil. Apply the oil directly to the skin cancer and cover it with a clean bandage. Re-apply fresh cannabis oil every 3 to 4 days as well as a new bandage. Continue treatment until the cancer is gone.

Once the cancer is gone continue to treat the same area where the cancer was for about two weeks. Doing this helps ensure that all the cancer cells die. If you've had skin cancer for a longer period of time it may take a longer time to cure. In most skin cancer cases the cancer disappears in less than three weeks. In extreme cases it could take longer. Just continue the treatment until the cancer is gone. The speed of healing all depends on your own rate of healing and how deep the cancer is.

You may find you dislike the taste of Cannabis oil especially at larger dosages. If so, I recommend you invest in #3 empty veggie gel capsules. With the Now brand #3's you can measure a 1/4 gram easily. You just fill it to almost full. A digital scale that measures down to 1/100th of a gram would be ideal to measure your first capsule but once you attain that 1/4 gram dose you can eyeball your capsules from there. You will need that scale while you are building up your dosage. Nine mills of cannabis oil is equal to one gram.

Cannabis Extracts

Cannabis contains over four hundred medicinal compounds, which create a beneficial synergy and becomes greater then the sum of its parts. Meaning they work together to enhance or inhibit endocannabinoid activity and there effects on the mind and body.

Cannabis is a herb and the essential oil extracted from the plant can be three to four times more potent when metabolized thru the gastric system.

Be careful when making or buying extracts. The finished product should be a thick tar like substance. If the oil is too thin it contains water or alcohol. Oh, and it might be illegal in your country.

Delta 9-Terahydrocannabinoil (THC)

9-tetrahydrocannabinoil (THC) ingested orally undergoes "first pass metabolism" in the small intestine and liver forming 11-hydroxy THC; the metabolite is more psychoactive than THC. Inhaled THC undergoes little first-pass metabolism, so less 11-hydroxy THC is formed. Smoking cannabis is an expedient in fighting fatigue, headache and exhaustion where as oral ingestion of cannabis results mostly as a narcotic effect. THC-9 boils at 157°C and its properties are Euphoriant, Analgesic, Anti-inflammatory, Antioxidant and Antiemetic.

Cannabinoil (CBD)

Cannabidiol (CBD) is the next-best studied phytocannabinoid after THC. CBD works in synergy with other compounds as a regulator.
CBD provides antipsychotic benefits. It increases dopamine activity, serves as a serotonin uptake inhibitor and enhances norepinephrine activity. CBD protects neurons from glutamate toxicity and serves as an antioxidant. THC inhibits receptor activity in the hippocampus and effects short-term memory. There is good reason for this but CBD on the other hand does not dampen the firing of hippocampal cells and does not disrupt learning. CBD works in synergy with other cannabinoids and is more effective medicinally then THC alone. CBD is non-psychoactive and has little effect on the immune system. CBD boils between 160-180°C. and its properties include Anxiolytic, Analgesic, Antipsychotic, Anti-inflammatory, Antioxidant and Antispasmodic.

Cannabinoil (CBN)

Cannabinol (CBN) is the degradation product of THC. CBN potentiates the effects of THC, which is why marijuana that has been well cured is more potent.

CBN boils at 185°C and its properties are Oxidation, breakdown, product, Sedative and Antibiotic.

Cannabigerol (CBG)

Cannabigerol (CBG) works in synergy with other cannabinoids and does more or less what other cannabinoids do but CBG has far superior anti bacterial and anti fungal properties. CBC boils at 220°C and is Anti-inflammatory, Antibiotic and Antifungal.

Terpenoids

The unique smell of cannabis arises from over one hundred terpenoid compounds. Terpenoids act on receptors and neurotransmitters as a serotonin uptake inhibitor. Terpenoids enhance norepinephrine activity, increase dopamine activity and augment GABA receptors.

Inhaling these synergistic terpenoids reduces anxiety and depression, which improves immune function via the neuroendocrine system by damping the hypothalamic-pituitary-adrenal axis.

Inhalation of terpenoids reduces the secretion of stress hormones and is very sedative. Inhaling terpenoids increases cerebral blood flow and enhances cortical activity.

Terpenoids are very effective at treating Alzheimer's disease.

Terpenoids boil between 119-224°C. There properties are Analgesic, Anti-inflamatory, Cytoprotective, Antimalarial, Cannabinoid agonist, Immune potentiator, Antidepresent, Antimutagenic, Sedative, Anxiolytic, Immune potentiator, Antipyretic, Increases cerebral blood flow, Stimulant, Antviral, Antinociceptive and Brochodilator.

Flavonoids

Flavonoids are aromatic, polycyclic phenols. Cannabis consists of about one percent flavonoids. Flavonoids have a wide range of biological effects including many properties found in terpenoids and cannabinoids. Flavonoids have a high affinity for estrogen receptors. Flavonoids boil between 134°-250°C. Flavonoids properties include Anxiolytic, Anti-inflammatory, Estrogenic, Anti-oxident, Antimutagenic, Antiviral and Antineoplastic.

Click on the link to view a video on Cannabis Extracts.

Cannabis Extracts

How To Make Cannabis Oil

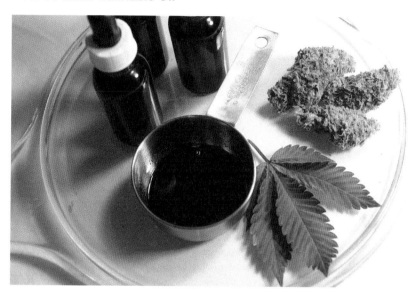

Making Cannabis Oil is easy but dangerous if you do not follow procedure.

By far the cleanest and safest method is CO2 extraction but unless you are mass-producing, the cost of equipment is unjustifiable. The next cleanest method is the dry ice method, which most people can do at home with minimal equiptment.

The most common form of extraction is to use alcohol and what type of alcohol to use is in high debate. What you need is pure alcohol, 95-99%. If you use Isopropyl, make sure it is not denatured, make sure it is unadulterated to prevent you from drinking it. If you use grain alcohol then Everclear 190 proof contains 95% alcohol. If Everclear is unavailable in your area, 180 proof Vodka or Rum will work.

Whatever alcohol you choose, make sure you follow procedure and ensure you have vaporized all of the alcohol before consuming it.

Alcohol has a saturation point of one gram of cannabis to six mills of alcohol, so when I make cannabis oil, I use two ounces of cannabis to five hundred mills of alcohol. This formula can be scaled up or down.

Grind your herb course.

For a narcotic effect, decarboxylate the cannabis in the oven at two hundred degrees for fifteen to twenty minutes.

After the herb cools down, put the cannabis in the freezer until frozen. This will help release the trichomes, which is the crystal that forms on the bud and leaf.

Drench the cannabis in alcohol. Use glass or stainless steel containers. Avoid using anything plastic.

Soak your herb in the alcohol, stir for a few minutes and strain the alcohol thru a wire mesh.

Strain the alcohol a second time thru a coffee filter.

Once the mix is strained, reduce the alcohol in a distiller, or a rice cooker. This is to be done out side with ventilation. Do not let anyone tell you it is save to do this indoors.

It won't take long to reduce and just as the oil begins to get thicker, you add a few drops of water. Since alcohol boils at a lower temperature then water it will burn off first ensuring all toxins have been purged from the oil.

When the oil becomes thick like paste, put it in a smaller container and finish it off on a plate warmer. When the oil stops bubbling the oil is save to consume.

The finished product should be of a tar like consistency when cooled down. You should yield seven grams of cannabis oil from two ounces of cannabis.

A note of caution, it is impossible to remove 100% of the alcohol. Trace amounts are left behind but it is not enough to cause any serious damage unless you use cannabis oil over extended periods of time. Cannabis Oil is a medication that is intended to treat a patient over a fixed period of time. It is not intended to be incorporated into someone's every day life style. When you are treating cancer, the benefits far out way the risk, plus the body has this amazing ability to flush toxins out of the body.

My argument about using isopropyl alcohol over ethanol alcohol that you buy from the liquor store is that isopropyl will convert to acetone after it is consumed and ethanol will convert into formaldehyde after consumption. The difference between the two is acetone is less toxic then formaldehyde, even though isopropyl is more toxic then ethanol alcohol.

I recommend you watch my Cannabis Oil video on YouTube before you attempt this. Here is the link.

Cannabis Oil Revised addition.

Cannabis Butter

Canna Butter is very popular. Animal fat contrary to popular believe is healthy for you, especially if you remove the milk solids by clarifying the butter. Animal fat is also ideal for fusing cannabinoids since cannabinoids are fat-soluble.

Thanks to large corporations and their influence on governments, vegetable fats have been marketed as a healthier choice over animal fat and the opposite is true.

The body, needs saturated fat, it prevents heart disease. On the other hand polyunsaturated fats from vegetable oils promotes heart disease. One hundred years ago before we started using vegetable oils, heart disease was virtually unknown.

Proctor and Gamble was the first to start marketing Crisco as a new kind of food, which they used originally to make soap and candles. The introduction of electricity lowered the demand for candles so Procter and Gamble decided to promote the fat as a healthier, all-vegetable-derived shortening and the onslaught of heart disease began.

Recent studies have proven that saturated fats lowers mortality rates and heart disease, so start consuming animal fats and stop using vegetable fats. Make soap, or candles out of vegetable fat but don't put it in your mouth and eat it.

Our government today still promotes vegetable fat as a healthier choice and they also promote saturated fat as an unhealthy choice to encourage us to consume less saturated fat and more polyunsaturated fat.

The government has a vested interest in the farming and production of vegetable oils and the medical community has done nothing but profit from this misinformation or should I say counter intelligence.

Now that you know the truth, take health care into your own hands. Let food be thy medicine and let medicine be thy food.

How To Make Cannabis Butter

Decarboxylate 28 gr of marijuana. You can use bud shake or a mix of the two. Place one pound of unsalted butter into a pot with four cups of water. Bring to a slow boil and melt the butter with the water.

Add 28 gr of coarsely grinded marijuana and cook for two to five hours. You may need to cook the cannabis for up to five hours if you are making larger batches.

Cannabinoids are released into the water and because cannabinoids are fat soluble, cannabinoids will attach to the butter. Make sure you don't boil off all the water. The water acts as a buffer and prevents the butter from exceeding 212° F.

When the butter is ready, remove from the heat and let it cool down to room temperature before you put it in the fridge. It would help to poor it into a different container.

When the butter is solidified, remove from the fridge. Cut the butter up and remove from the water. Discard the water and clean any milk solids that have attached to the bottom of the butter. It helps to clarify the butter first.

Your butter is now ready for consumption, cooking or baking. Enjoy.

28g times 1000 equals 28,000 mg of dry weight times 14% THC equals 3920 mg of THC. divided by approximately 600ml of coconut oil equals 6.53mg of THC per 1ml of butter.

This is a potent recipe. You could easily scale it down for a milder butter or use shake.

Use up to 1ml of cannabis butter for each portion your recipe yields. Just simply substitute a portion of the fat in your recipe with cannabis butter. If you baked a dozen cookies or muffins you would use 12ml of cannabis butter in the recipe.

Check out my YouTube channel or my website for instructional videos on how to make Canna Butter.

Canna Butter

Coconut Oil

The health benefits of coconut oil include hair care, skin care, stress relief. cholesterol level maintenance, weight loss, balanced immune system, digestion and regulated metabolism. It also provides relief from kidney problems, heart diseases, high blood pressure, diabetes, HIV, and cancer while helping to improve dental quality and bone strength.

The benefits of coconut oil can be attributed to the presence of lauric acid, capric acid and caprylic acid and their respective properties, such as antimicrobial, antioxidant, anti-fungal and antibacterial.

Coconut oil is used extensively in tropical countries, especially India, Sri Lanka, Thailand, Philippines, etc. At one time, the oil was also popular in western countries like the United States and Canada. There was a strong propaganda campaign in the seventies, spread by the corn oil and soy oil industry against coconut oil. Coconut oil was considered harmful for the human body due to its high saturated fat content until the last decade when people began to question the claims of the corporate propaganda machine.

How lauric acid is used by the body

The human body converts lauric acid into monolaurin, which is helpful in dealing with viruses and bacteria that cause diseases such as herpes, influenza, cytomegalovirus and even HIV.

Coconut Oil

More than ninety percent of coconut oil consists of saturated fats, along with traces of unsaturated fatty acids, such as monounsaturated fatty acids and polyunsaturated fatty acids.

Saturated fatty acids.

Most of them are medium chain triglycerides, which assimilate well in the body's systems and is perfect for fusing cannabis. Lauric acid is the chief contributor, representing more than forty percent of the total, followed by capric acid, caprylic acid, myristic acid and palmitic.

There is a misconception spread among many people that coconut oil is not good for heart health. This is because it contains a large quantity of saturated fats. In reality, coconut oil is beneficial for the heart. It contains about 50% lauric acid, which helps in actively preventing various heart problems, like high cholesterol levels and high blood pressure.

The saturated fats present in coconut oil are not harmful, as you commonly find in vegetable oils. Coconut oil does not lead to an increase in LDL levels and it reduces the incidence of injury and damage to arteries and therefore helps in preventing atherosclerosis.

Healing and Infections

Coconut oil is recommended for many health benefits that are explained below.

Liver: The presence of medium chain triglycerides and fatty acids helps in preventing liver diseases because coconut oil is easily converted into energy when they reach the liver, thus reducing the work load of the liver and preventing accumulation of fat.

Kidney: Coconut oil helps prevent kidney and gall bladder diseases. It also helps to dissolve kidney stones.

Pancreatitis: Coconut oil is also useful in treating pancreatitis.

Stress relief: Coconut oil is very soothing and hence it helps in removing stress. Applying coconut oil followed by a gentle massage, helps to eliminate fatigue.

Diabetes: Coconut oil helps in controlling blood sugar and improves the secretion of insulin. It also promotes the utilization of blood glucose, thereby preventing and treating diabetes.

Bones: Coconut oil improves the ability of our body to absorb minerals. These include calcium and magnesium, which are necessary for the development of bones. Thus, coconut oil is very useful to those who are prone to osteoporosis after middle age.

Dental care: Calcium is an important component for healthy teeth. Coconut oil facilitates absorption of calcium by the body. Coconut oil develops strong teeth and stops tooth decay.

HIV and cancer: It is believed that coconut oil reduces a person's viral susceptibility for HIV and cancer patients. Research has shown an indication of this effect of coconut oil on reducing the viral load of HIV patients.

Coconut oil is used by athletes and those who are dieting. Coconut oil contains fewer calories than other oils, its fat content is easily converted into energy and it does not lead to an accumulation of fat in the heart and arteries. Coconut oil helps boost energy, endurance and enhances the performance of athletes.

Coconut oil and Alzheimer's disease: Research conducted by Dr. Newport states that coconut oil is useful in treating Alzheimer's disease. There is no scientific evidence or traditional knowledge of coconut oil being used for treating Alzheimer's

Why is coconut oil solid: Coconut oil has a high melting point, about 76-78° F. Therefore it is solid at room temperature. If you buy a bottle of coconut oil and find it solid, don't assume there is a problem with it. Coconut oil is often in this form.

Coconut canna oil is probably the healthiest medicated food in existence. I do not recommend you use any other oil. Coconut oil is a medium chain fatty acid and is perfect for cannabinoid fusion. Coconut oil contains 90% saturated fat and 50% fatty acids and is very good for our health. It is also a non-GMO food.

Canna oil is not to be confused with cannabis oil or hemp oil.

How to make Canna Coconut Oil

Decarboxylate 28 g of cannabis.

Grind in a blender. Course, not fine.

Wrap Cannabis in a double layer of cheesecloth.

Freeze the cannabis for two to three hours then place the cannabis in a slow cooker on low with 400 ml of organic coconut oil.

Cook for four-five hours stirring occasionally, turn off heat and let it cool for one hour.

Remove the cannabis and squeeze the coconut oil out of the cheesecloth by twisting it.

Cool down to room temperature before storing in the fridge. Store for as long as the coconut oil is good for. Coconut oil has a long shelve life, around two years.

This is a very potent recipe if you use all bud. You could use shake and still end up with very potent coconut oil. If you started out with herb that is 14% THC. 1 ml of olive oil will contain 9.8 mg of THC.

A little will go along way in your recipes. You could easily scale this recipe down to 3 gr of bud or 6 gr of sugar shake to 400 ml of coconut oil. You would end up with 1.05 mg of THC to 1 ml of coconut oil. 5 ml equals a teaspoon and would contain 5.25 mg of THC. 3 gr of bud is 3000 mg time's 14 % THC content, which equals 420 mg of THC divided by 400 ml of coconut oil.
Check out my YouTube channel or my website for instructional videos on how to make Canna Oil.

28,000 ml times 14% THC equals 3920 mg of THC divided by 400 ml of coconut oil equals 9.8 mg. of THC to one ml of oil.

Cannabis Coconut Oil

Canna Oil

Dosage Information

The FDA recommends 5-10 mg per 100 kg of body weight as a single dosage of THC. Start on a mild dosage and wait until you feel the effects of the medication before you increase your dosage. It usually takes at least one hour before you start to feel the effects so be patient. It could take up to two hours.

Cannabis Infused Olive Oil

Decarboxylate 2 grams of bud or 4 grams of sugar shake. Coarse grind your herb and roll it up in a double layer of cheesecloth. Don't pack it too tight. Bring the herb to a boil in 3 cups of water and 1 cup of olive oil. Keep the temperature low, at a slow rolling boil. Be sure not to boil off the water. Cook for one hour and let it cool down to room temperature. Remove the herb wrapped in cheesecloth, squeeze and twist until you have drained off most of the olive oil.

Pour the water and olive oil into a bowl and place it in the freezer until the olive oil has solidified. Drain the water from the solidified oil and place the oil in a different container for storage. Make small amounts, cooked olive oil will go rancid fast. Store in the fridge in an airtight container.

2 grams of herb is equal to 2,000 milligrams, times 14%(average THC content) equals 280 milligrams of THC in 8oz. of olive oil, which equals 236.588 milliliters. 280 milligrams of THC divided by 236.588 milliliters equals 1.18 milligrams of THC in a milliliter of olive oil. One teaspoon of olive oil will contain approximately 5.9 milligrams of THC.

You could use more herb and make the olive oil more potent or less herb and make it less potent. Less is more. You can make potent cannabis olive oil with just sugar shake. I would save the bud for other things.

Cannabis Paste

The ancients made cannabis paste over four thousand years ago. They used to bathe in it. When cannabis paste is absorbed by the skin it enters the blood stream. Some claim cannabis paste is more effective then Hash Oil and after using it myself I would tend to agree.

The ancients used to put cannabis in a ceramic pot with coconut oil or olive oil. Cover it with a lid and leave it in the hot sun for three or four days.

I have developed a more practical method achieving good results in twelve hours of cooking at low temperatures.

Grind up one ounce of marijuana. You can use leaf, bud, sugar shake or a mix of the three ingredients. There is more CBD in the leaf then there is in the bud so formulating a recipe that works for you is in your control. Grind the cannabis into a flour and strain it thru a cake sifter.

Place the cannabis in a mason jar with 125ml of coconut oil. I recommend coconut oil over olive oil because it can go rancid fast after heat is applied. Place in a water bath and cook for 10-12 hours. The lower the temperature and the longer the cooking time the better.

Some people have placed it in a dark warm cupboard in the kitchen for a few months.

Once the paste is cooled down it can be stored in the fridge for as long as the coconut oils shelve life or up to two months.
I have found it more effective then hash oil for my skin condition. I rub it into my skin and there is definitely greater effect with the paste.

It doesn't taste very good so if you plan on ingesting paste, gel caps might be the way to go. Cooking with paste will only deteriorate your medication so eating it raw in gel caps is more effective. You can decarboxylate your herb for that narcotic effect or you can keep temperatures below 175°F. By doing this you do not activate the cannabinoids in the herb and you are able to increase the dosage without increasing the narcotic effect.

Here is a link to my video on how to make Cannabis Paste.

Cannabis Paste

Cannabis Cream

Cannabis cream is a natural organic moisturizer that rejuvenates the skin. Cannabis Cream is made from Cannabis Coconut Oil or organic Hemp Oil, bees wax and filtered water.

Everything you put on your skin is absorbed by your skin and ends up in your blood stream. In essence your skin eats everything you put on it. Cannabis Cream is an effective way of consuming cannabinoids because it avoids the gastric system.

Hemp Oil has the health benefits of Marijuana but without the psychoactive effects of THC. Hemp oil contains large amounts of CBD and other cannnabinoids grown from cannabis sativa strains with a THC content of less then 0.3%. Hemp oil is legal and safe to use.

Cannabis Cream helps regenerate the skin's protective layer. Thanks to its content of Omega 3 and Omega 6 fatty acids, like hemp oil has a composition similar to skin lipids which makes it an excellent natural emollient and moisturizer. It is an ingredient in many skin and body care products. Hemp oil helps to calm irritated skin.

Cannabis Hemp Cream energizes the skin. Moisturizing, regenerating and revitalizing, cannabis cream is especially useful for dry, tired or dehydrated skin. Skin regeneration and hydration of dry mature skin are enhanced through the use of Cannabis Cream and hemp oil. It increases the skins elasticity and water retention capacity in tissues.

Hemp oil has the ideal combination of fatty acids. Hemp oil is the only vegetable oil that contains Omega 3 and Omega 6 fatty acids in the ideal ratio of 3 to 1 for optimal body needs.

Place one cup of cannabis coconut oil in a bowl over a water bath and add one ounce of bees wax. Heat until the bees wax is melted, around 145°F. You can add essential oils to scent the cream or utilize its health properties at this point. Allow the mix to cool down and blend in one cup of filtered water. You can fuse marijuana into the water if desired. Other herbs can be use too but you have to know what you are doing about that.
Use a hand held mixer. Add the water slowly and the more water you add the thicker it will get. That's it. Store in a sterilized food grade container, not plastic.

Cannabis Cream should keep for two weeks unrefrigerated and up to two months in the fridge.

Here is a link to my video on how to make Cannabis Cream.

Cannabis Cream

Hemp Cream

Hemp Cream is a brand new product that I am working on and will be launched in the very near future. It is made the way I make Cannabis Cream only I replace the coconut cannabis oil with hemp oil. It is not just a natural organic skin moisturizer. It is edible and it can also be used as a lubricant. The viscosity of hemp oil is bar none.

For more information on the product please check out my website.

http://hempcream.co

Tinctures

Tinctures are easy to prepare. They are effective and discrete. Tinctures are not new. Until cannabis was banned in 1937, tinctures were the primary type of cannabis medicines. Tinctures are essentially alcohol extractions of cannabis, usually bud and shake. Tinctures are easy to make and very inexpensive. Tinctures contain all 70-80 of the essential cannabinoids instead of only one with Marinol. Like most pharmaceutical drugs, they come with harmful side effects including death.

Some of the cannabinoids such as cannibidiol (CBD) actually reduce the psychoactive effects of THC while increasing the overall efficacy of the preparation.

The best way to use tinctures is under the tongue. Dosage control is easily achieved by the number of drops a patient places under the tongue, where the medicine is rapidly absorbed into the arterial system and is quickly absorbed into the blood stream. All a patient has to do with tinctures is use a few drops and wait for the effects and either use more or stop as the situation indicates.

Tinctures can be flavored for better taste. They are best stored in dark bottles in the refrigerator. Since tinctures average 75% alcohol there is little worry of bacterial, or other biological contamination.

Tinctures are designed to address the problems of rapid medicine delivery and consistent dosing. Most tinctures are to be used under the tongue. Absorption by the arterial blood supply under the tongue is completed in seconds. One trick is to not swallow the dose as, if swallowed, absorption will be in the GI tract. Many patients though add their tincture to a cup of tea, coffee or juice for easy delivery. When tinctures are used in a beverage, absorption will be slower than if absorbed under the tongue. Usually, a tincture dose is delivered by means of a medicine dropper or a teaspoon. A rule of thumb on dosage is that patients receive benefit from 3-4 drops to a couple of full droppers, depending upon the potency of the tincture and the patient's own requirements.

The method listed below will detail the methods of preparing a tincture. While the methods are optimized for purity and potency, ultimately these will largely be determined by the purity and potency of the cannabis from which the tincture is made. Another item of note in regard to starting material for tinctures is the selection of strain. Trial and error is usually required to acquire the appropriate strain and the proper dose level.

General Rules

Tinctures are an extraction of active cannabinoids from plant material. Cannabis contains many chemicals that can either upset the stomach or taste nasty. One of the goals of extraction is to secure the cannabinoids while leaving the chlorophylls as much as possible.

Both heat and light adversely effect cannabinoids and should be avoided or minimized. Tinctures should be stored in airtight dark glass containers, kept at cool temperatures. Avoid plastic containers. The alcohol will solubilize some of the free vinyl's in the plastic.

Cold Method (recommended)

Here is a recipe for a high quality tincture. This method does not use heat so it keeps the integrity of the cannabinoids intact.

Decarboxylate four grams of cannabis, you can use a combination of bud and shake depending on your needs. Grind coarse and place in a mason jar with four ounces of Bacardi 151 proof. You can also use a high proof Vodka, or Everclear if it is available. Seal the lid and shake periodically, keep in a dark cool place. A good tincture can be achieved in a few minutes contrary to popular believe. Some people take days if not weeks or months to do this but it actually only takes minutes to extract cannabinoids from alcohol. The longer you take, the more chlorophyll you will extract, making the tincture bitter.

Tinctures are increasing in popularity because tinctures are easy to prepare and very effective. You can use tinctures with just about anything. I use a few drops in my coffee. The heat will burn off most of the alcohol.

Check out my YouTube channel or my website for an instructional video on how to make tinctures.

Cannabis Tinctures

Cannabis Root

Cannabis root contains very high levels of CBD, which makes it a very valuable medicine. There are many ways that it can be prepared. It can be dried out and ground into flour. From there you can make paste or salves. It can be also consumed raw. It can also be juiced or added to smoothies. You can also make tea out of the dried root.

Cannabis root was used extensively as a medicine by the ancients. It is also used to counteract the effects of THC. If you under estimate an edible or you just loose control and get the munchies, cannabis root can be used to counter act the effects of THC. Cannabis (the dried, cured flower we know as bud can contain very little CBD when tested. Cannabis root can be used to fortify your infusions and extractions. The root could also be used to regulate levels of THC in your medicine.

Add 2 tsp. of cannabis root to a smoothie and wait for about an hour for it to kick in. Your pain will melt away leaving you feeling relaxed without a heavy THC buzz. You will feel perfectly medicated for most of the day feeling energetic, happy and feeling good for daytime activities.

In much of the world, the main methods of preparation have been consistent through time. The root is either applied raw, dried, boiled, soaked, roasted or occasionally reduced to ash. The ancients believe that cannabis root ash and honey can rejuvenate hair growth when applied to the scalp.

If boiled for a short time it can be drunk as a tea, if boiled for a longer time it reduces to a thick, dark extract resembling pitch or heavy oil. If it is dried or roasted and ground, it forms a powder that can be rendered into salves or poultices; soaking it can produce a soothing, moist bandage for inflamed, burned or irritated skin.

Poultices

A poultice is made by mashing plant material with warm water or natural oils to make a paste. The paste can be applied directly to the skin and covered with a clean cloth. The cloth can then be covered in plastic wrap to retain moisture. Change the poultice every three to four hours or whenever it dries out.

Compresses

A compress is used the same way but warm liquids are applied to the cloth instead of raw substances. Tinctures or herbal infusions are great for compresses

Salves

Beeswax is a wonderful, natural ingredient you can use to make your own salves. On its own, beeswax isn't a moisturizer, but when mixed with other ingredients, such as Shea butter, coconut oil, olive oil, jojoba oil or other natural oils, beeswax acts as a moisture barrier on your skin, protecting it from drying out and allowing the oils in the salve to soak into your skin. A few drops of essential oil can be added to your salve mixture for scent or therapeutic purposes. You can also infuse oil with the herbs of your choice and use it in your salve mixture.

When choosing essential oils to add to your salve, it's important not to use ones that are phototoxic, they increase the skin's sensitivity to UV light and increase your risk of sunburn. Most citrus-based essential oils are phototoxic. Other essential oils that could be a problem include angelica, bergamot, cumin, dill, tagetes and yuzu.

Essential oils have unique properties. Here are some examples of just a few.

Rosemary: helps relieve tired muscles
Tea tree: antiseptic properties
Eucalyptus: relieves congestion
Lavender: antiseptic and calming properties
Peppermint: helps relieve tired muscles and congestion

A general rule of thumb when making salves is to use one part bees wax to three to five parts oil. If you are unhappy with the consistency of your finished salve, you can adjust the ratios of beeswax to oil. More beeswax makes a thicker, more solid salve, while less beeswax gives the salve a creamier consistency.

Oils useful for moisturizing and mixing with beeswax are listed below.

- **Jojoba oil** is an excellent moisturizing oil. Use it sparingly. One ounce of jojoba oil is usually enough for a salve mix.
- **Almond oil** is another good moisturizing oil, but you should avoid it if you have sensitivities or allergies to nuts.
- **Olive oil** has been used as a moisturizer since ancient times. It contains many antioxidants and won't clog pores. It does go rancid fast which greatly reduces its shelve life.
- **Coconut oil** also has been used as a moisturizer for centuries. Be sure to purchase virgin coconut oil, which isn't processed with harsh chemicals. I highly recommend coconut oil for the many reasons that I have mentioned in this book.
- **Hemp oil** is also an excellent choice for salves. Even though hemp oil contains CBD it lacks the THC to create synergy. It is less effective as a medicine but great as a supplement or a moisturizer with many health benefits.

Directions

To make a salve you first must infuse your cannabis root into oil. I personally prefer coconut oil. Just simply add cannabis root to the oil in a Mason jar and store in a warm dark place for several months. You can speed up the process by adding heat. Please refer to my canna coconut oil method for this or my Hemp or Cannabis Cream method.

Melt the beeswax in a double boiler, let cool slightly and blend in the oils. Pour Salve into tin or glass containers and let it cool over night before attaching the lids. The Salve should keep for three to four months in the fridge.

Cannabis root has been used medicinally for centuries from different parts of the world and to treat a wide range of ailments. The earliest report is from medieval times when the root was said to relieve the agonies of gout and other painful diseases.

Cannabis root is also used to treat tetanus, colic, gastralgia, swelling of the liver, gonorrhea, sterility, impotency, tuberculosis of the lungs and asthma.

Cannabis root has fallen by the waist side, thousands of pounds of valuable medicine is being thrown into the compost heap everyday. The cannabis revolution needs to get back to its roots and discover where the real medicine is. In the roots, the leaves, the stems as well as the bud. Whole plant medicine holistically restores physiological balance.

Sources

In1696 Georg Eberhard Rumpf (Rumphius), a German physician at the service of the Dutch Crown reported on the use of cannabis root in Indonesia to treat gonorrhea (Rumpf and Beekman 1981, Russo 2002). By 1763 The New English Dictionary said cannabis root applied to skin eases inflammation (Marijuana as Medicine 2005). In the Chinese Materia Medica "juice of the root is thought to have a beneficial action in retained placenta and post partum hemorrhage, (Stuart 1928).

In Argentina cannabis is considered a real panacea and is used to treat tetanus, colic, gastralgia, swelling of the liver, gonorrhea, sterility, impotency, abortion, tuberculosis of the lungs and asthma even the root-bark has been collected in spring, and employed as a febrifuge, tonic, for treatment of dysentery and gastralgia, either pulverized or in form of decoctions. The root when ground and applied to burns is said to relieve pain. Oil from the seeds has been frequently used even in treatment of cancer (Kabelik, 1960).

Cooking with Cannabis

Cooking with cannabis is easier then you think it is. Once you dive in and do some experimenting of your own, you will be cooking like a pro in no time.

Now that you have learned how to make infusions and extractions, it is time to start cooking. A big mistake people make when cooking with cannabis is that they cook off most of the cannabinoid content when using high temperatures. It is best to avoid high temperatures as much as possible, especially if you are using marijuana as medication.

Do not fast fry or panfry cannabis. Instead, add the cannabis at the end of the cooking process, after you turn down the heat. The cooling down process will draw cannabinoids out and help bind them to the fats in your food. The process is like steeping tea. I recommend using this procedure when cooking with extracts and infusions. It is the best way to preserve your cannabinoids.

With this method you can use cannabutter, cannaoil, hash, kief, cannabis oil, tinctures, wax and shatter.

Now that propane is available in food grade cans, wax and shatter have become less toxic and safer to use.

I would use this same method for making soups and sauces as well or wait until you have finished caramelizing your meats and vegetables. Soups and sauces will boil at 212ºF and cannabinoids start to break down at 220ºF.

Season your ingredients lightly in the beginning to enhance flavor but you should add your herbs and garlic or what ever other aromatics you are using at the end. This will preserve the nutritional and medicinal benefits of your food. Season to taste after your soup or sauce has reduced. Food is medicine.

This guide is about maintaining and restoring health and there are some foods you should avoid. Number one is sugar. Cut it out of your diet completely and do not eat foods that have sugar added to it. All food contain natural sugars, you don't need to add more. In time your taste buds will adjust to a more balanced diet.

Avoid using white flour, use whole-wheat flour instead. It is more nutritious but try to avoid eating to many carbohydrates and too much gluten.

The bulk of your diet should be fruits and vegetables. You really do not need allot of protein or carbohydrates in your diet. You can use plant based proteins like fresh raw marijuana, whole grains, seeds and legumes. Reduce the amount of meat in your diet.

Dairy products and vegetable fats should also be avoided.

Try to use organic ingredients and eat the food that is grown locally in your area.

Replace the table salt with sea salt.

Avoid eating processed food.

Avoid alcohol.

When making deserts and candy keep it simple. Honey and real maple syrup are great healthy alternatives for sugar.

Flavors like dark chocolate, coffee and raspberries work well in masking the flavor of hemp. Yuk...

Know your numbers

The idea is to make your infusions and extractions as potent as possible. This way you can use as little as possible in your recipe with not much effect on the taste of your finished product.

Be aware when ingesting cannabis, THC9 converts into THC11, which is more potent and longer lasting.

When calculating how much extract or infusion to use in your recipe, start out with how potent your herb was. If your herb had a THC content of 14% and you want to fuse 28 grams of marijuana into 454 grams of butter, convert the dry weight of your marijuana into milligrams. One gram of dry herb is equal to one thousand milligrams so 28 grams is equal to 28,000 milligrams times 14% is equal to 3920 milligrams of THC in 454 grams of butter. 3920 divided by 454 equals 8.634 milligrams of THC in a gram of canna butter. The FDA recommends 5-10 milligrams per 100 kilograms of body weight. For an average person I would say 3-7 milligrams is recommended but for first timers I would cut that in half or less and see how that goes. It can take up to two hours for your body to metabolize THC so be patient. Everyone's sensitivity is different and it is best to start small until you build up some tolerance.

Cannabis Chocolate

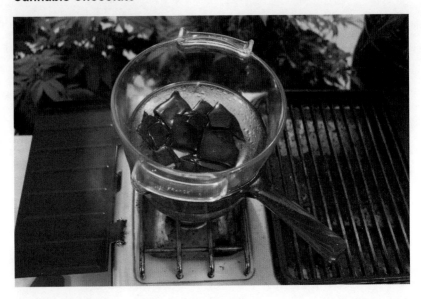

Canna chocolate is to be made with dark chocolate because of its fat content. Dark chocolate contains healthy saturated fat and because cannabinoids are fat soluble, they attach to the fat in the chocolate.

Dark chocolate is loaded with nutrients that can positively affect your health.

Made from the seed of the cocoa tree, it is one of the best sources of antioxidants in the world.

Studies show that dark chocolate can improve health and lower the risk of heart disease.

Dark Chocolate is Very Nutritious

Buy quality dark chocolate with a high cocoa content, it is very nutritious. It contains a decent amount of soluble fiber and is loaded with minerals.

A 100-gram bar of dark chocolate with 70-85% cocoa contains.

11 grams of fiber
67% of the RDA for Iron
58% of the RDA for Magnesium
89% of the RDA for Copper
98% of the RDA for Manganese

Dark chocolate also contains potassium, phosphorus, zinc and selenium.

100 grams (3.5 ounces) is a fairly large amount and not something you should be consuming daily. All these nutrients also come with 600 calories and small amounts of sugar. For these reasons, dark chocolate should be consumed in moderation.

The fatty acid profile of cocoa and dark chocolate is excellent. The fats are mostly saturated and monounsaturated, with small amounts of polyunsaturated fat.

It also contains stimulants like caffeine and theobromine, but is unlikely to keep you awake at night as the amount of caffeine is very small compared to coffee.

Quality dark chocolate is rich in Fiber, Iron, Magnesium, Copper, Manganese and a few other minerals.

Dark Chocolate is a Powerful Source of Antioxidants

Dark chocolate is loaded with organic compounds that are biologically active and function as antioxidants. These include polyphenols, flavanols, catechins, among others.
One study showed that cocoa and dark chocolate contained more antioxidant activity, polyphenols and flavanols than other fruits tested, which included blueberries and Acai berries.

Cocoa and dark chocolate have a wide variety of powerful antioxidants, way more than most other foods.

Dark Chocolate May Improve Blood Flow and Lower Blood Pressure

The flavanols in dark chocolate can stimulate the endothelium, the lining of arteries, to produce Nitric Oxide.

One of the functions of NO is to send signals to the arteries to relax, which lowers resistance to blood flow and therefore reduces blood pressure.

The bioactive compounds in cocoa can improve blood flow in the arteries and cause a small but statistically significant decrease in blood pressure.

Dark Chocolate Raises HDL and Protects LDL Against Oxidation

Consuming dark chocolate can improve several important risk factors for heart disease.

In a controlled trial, cocoa powder was found to significantly decrease oxidized LDL cholesterol. It also increased HDL and lowered total LDL with elevated cholesterol.

Oxidized LDL means that the LDL (bad cholesterol) has reacted with free radicals.
This makes the LDL particle itself reactive and capable of damaging other tissues, such as the lining of the arteries in your heart.

It makes perfect sense that cocoa lowers oxidized LDL. It contains an abundance of powerful antioxidants that do make it into the bloodstream and protect lipoproteins against oxidative damage.

Dark chocolate can also reduce insulin resistance, which is another common risk factor for many diseases like heart disease and diabetes.

Dark chocolate improves several important risk factors for disease. It lowers the susceptibility of LDL to oxidative damage while increasing HDL and improving insulin sensitivity.

Dark Chocolate May Lower The Risk of Cardiovascular Disease

The compounds in dark chocolate appear to be highly protective against the oxidation of LDL.

In the long term, this should cause much less cholesterol to lodge in the arteries and we should see a lower risk of heart disease over the long term.

It turns out that we have several long-term observational studies that show a fairly drastic improvement.

In a study of 470 elderly people, cocoa was found to reduce the risk of cardiovascular death by a whopping 50% over a 15 year period.

Another study revealed that eating chocolate 2 or more times per week lowered the risk of having calcified plaque in the arteries by 32%. Eating chocolate less frequently had no effect.

Another study showed that chocolate 5+ times per week lowered the risk of cardiovascular disease by 57%.

Dark Chocolate May Improve Brain Function

One study of healthy volunteers showed that 5 days of consuming high-flavanol cocoa improved blood flow to the brain.

Cocoa may also significantly improve cognitive function in people with mental impairment. It also improves verbal fluency and several risk factors for disease.

Cocoa also contains stimulant substances like caffeine and theobromine, which may be a key reason cocoa can improve brain function in the short term.

Dark chocolate also contains several chemical compounds that have a positive effect on your mood and cognitive health. Chocolate contains phenyl ethylamine, the same chemical your brain creates when you feel like you're falling in love. PEA encourages your brain to release endorphins, so eating dark chocolate will make you feel happier and is probably why I love dark chocolate.

Now that we know how beneficial dark chocolate is for our health and how ideal it is for cannabis infusion, it makes sense to use it as a power food and a medication. After all food is nature's pharmacy.

How to make Canna Chocolate

Heat up 100 grams of dark chocolate in a double boiler. Use a dark chocolate that has a high percentage of cocoa.

Weigh 10 grams of cannabis and decarboxylate if THC is an important factor in your medication.

Grind up the herb and freeze for about an hour. This helps release the trichomes from the cannabis.

Add melted chocolate to the cannabis and stir. This only takes a few minutes. You can add coconut or a natural extract like mint to mask the flavor of the cannabis. This is optional.

Pour the Cannabis Chocolate into molds or on wax paper and let it cool until hardened.

Your Canna Chocolate is now ready for consumption.

For an instructional video on how to make Canna Chocolate please visit my website or my YouTube channel.

Canna Chocolate

Cannabis Chocolate Dosage Information

Ten grams of chocolate will contain one gram of Cannabis and I consider that a heavy dosage. Start with a mild dosage of approximately three grams of chocolate and wait for about an hour before increasing your dosage. If you have a slow metabolism, it could take up to two hours before you feel the effects of the medication, so be patient.

Mashoon Hash

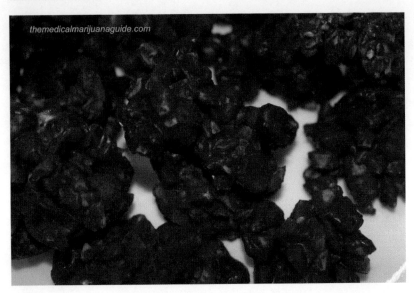

themedicalmarijuanaguide.com

Mashoon is an ancient recipe originating from Morocco. The recipe uses power foods like mixed nuts, dried fruit, dark chocolate, coconut oil, honey, butter and hashish.

This recipe is very effective as a medicine because it is a no bake recipe so most of the cannabinoids are preserved. The ancients knew what they where doing.

Ingredients

100 gr. mixed nuts
100 gr. dried fruit
100 gr. dark chocolate
1 tbs. honey
1tbs coconut oil
1 tbs. butter
A pinch of sea salt
Spices
1.5 gr. hash
Heat the butter and the coconut oil to 220º F. Add the hash and decarboxylate for 15-20 minutes. Add the dark chocolate, honey, salt and spices. You can use

cinnamon, cloves, all spice or what ever. Stir until well blended. Place dried fruit and nuts in a bowl and blend in the chocolate.

Weigh out 10 gr portions.

Let the mix cool down to room temperature and place in the fridge for 30 minutes until the chocolate has solidified.

Enjoy.

Here is a link to my video on how to make Mashoon.

Mashoon Hash

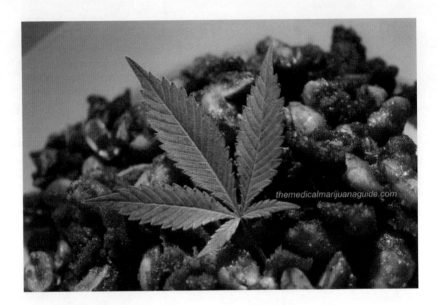

Peanut Hash Brittle

Hmmm. It was so good I forgot how to make it. Fortunately I made a video on it. The link to my YouTube channel is at the back of my book.

I do not recommend Peanut Hash Brittle as a steady medication. The sugar creates an imbalance but I feel it is ok to indulge once in awhile. The body has this amazing ability to heal itself if you feed it right.

My family makes Peanut Brittle once a year to celebrate on special occasions. They do not put any cannabis in it but it is something we all look forward too.

The recipe is coming to me. I will give it to you but you didn't get it from me ok. Sugar bad.
I upgraded the traditional recipe by replacing GMO foods with organic foods like cane sugar instead of beat sugar and maple syrup instead of corn syrup. Corn is very acid forming and it is virtually indigestible.

Ingredients

½ cup of water
1 cup of raw cane sugar
½ cup of maple syrup

1 tbs. butter
1 tsp. vanilla extract
1 cup of peanuts
1/8 tsp. sea salt
1 tsp. baking soda
3 gr. Hash

Ok let's see if I can remember how to do this.

Melt the butter and the hash in a small pan. You don't really need to decarboxylate it. Keep the temperature below 175°F.

In a separate pot add water, sugar and bring to a boil. Boil until the syrup reaches the crack stage, around 300°F. Add sea salt and stir to avoid burning.

Place a lid on the pot to prevent the sugar from crystalizing. Once the syrup comes to a boil you can add the maple syrup. Add the peanuts and stir being careful not to burn the peanuts.

When the syrup reaches the crack stage turn off the heat and stir in the butter and the hash and the vanilla extract.

Pour mix onto a tray lined with parchment paper and let it cool down before you put it in the fridge.

Do I have to tell you not to touch it, it's freaking hot, man.

After it has cooled down in the fridge you can break it up and eat it.

It will hit you in about an hour or two.

I would personally advise you to wait until the mix cools down to below 220°F before you add the butter and hash. If you do, you run the risk of crystalizing the sugar.
Above is a picture of my peanut hash brittle crystalized. It worked much better as a medication that way.

My second batch that didn't crystalize lost a lot of pow in its punch.

There you have it.

Peanut Hash Brittle ready for consumption.

Here is the link to my YouTube video on how to make Mashoon Hash. Don't forget to subscribe.

<u>Mashoon Hash</u>

Cannabis Cookies

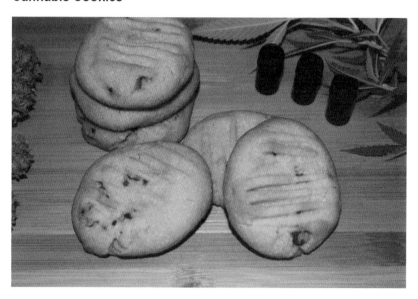

Chocolate Chip

Ingredients

1 cup of unsalted cannabutter, room temperature
1 1/2 cups light brown sugar
1/2 cup granulated sugar
1 tsp. vanilla extract
1 large egg, room temperature
2 cups all-purpose flour
1/2 tsp. baking soda
1/2 tsp. salt
11/2 cups dark chocolate chips

Procedure

Pre heat oven to 375ºF and line cookie trays with parchment paper.
Place butter and sugar in a mixing bowl and blend on medium speed until butter is creamed. This procedure incorporates air. Blend in the vanilla extract then blend in the egg.

In a separate bowl mix together the dry ingredients and blend into the butter and sugar at low speed until just blended. Do not over work the dough. Stir in the chocolate chips.

Use 2 tbsp. portions and place on a prepared cookie sheet 3 inches apart.

Bake for 6-7 minutes or until the edges are golden brown. Let cookies cool slightly before placing on a cooling rack.
The recipe will yield around 24 cookies. Once cooled, store in an airtight container for up to a week.

Chocolate Brownies

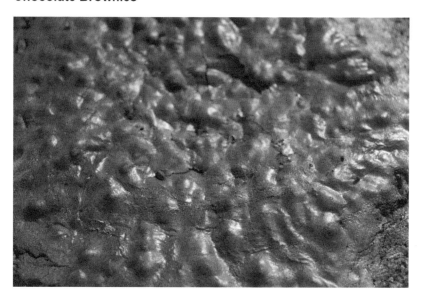

Ingredients

1/2 cup cannabutter
1 cup white sugar
2 eggs
1 tsp. vanilla extract
1/3 cup cocoa powder
1/2 cup all purpose flour
1/4 tsp. sea salt
1/4 tsp. baking powder

Frosting
3 tbs. cannabutter
3 tbs. cocoa powder
1 tbs. honey
1 tsp. vanilla extract
1 cup confectioners sugar

Procedure

pre heat oven to 350°F and grease and flour baking pans.

In a large saucepan melt 1/2 cup of cannabutter and remove from heat. Stir in sugar, eggs and 1 tsp. of vanilla extract. Beat in 1/3 cup of cocoa, 1/2 cup of flour, salt and baking powder. Pour batter into prepared pans and bake for 25 to 30 minutes.

To make the frosting mix 3 tbs. of softened cannabutter, 3 tbs. of cocoa, honey, 1 tsp. of vanilla extract and 1 cup of confectioners sugar. Mix until smooth. Frost the brownies while they are still warm.

Hemp Milk

Hemp Milk is a power food. Made from marijuana hemp seed, containing less then 0.30% THC. This is not enough to get you high.

Hemp seed is a complete protein with ten amino fatty acids. The proteins digest easily. Hemp is a quick source of food energy and is an abundant source of fibre, vitamins, minerals and nutrition.

Ancient civilizations have evolved entirely around the marijuana plant as a source of food, fuel and medicine. Hemp Milk is an excellent substitute for cows milk. I have been led to believe by the corporate propaganda machine that cows milk is a beneficial food but the truth behind all that marketing, promoting and corporate science is a fast track to cancer and heart disease.

Cows milk is breast milk and we are the only species on earth who drinks breast milk in adulthood, plus we are the only species on earth who will drink breast milk from another species. The reason for this is because breast milk is for babies who need a rich source of fat, protein and nutrition. Proteins from breast milk bypass the gastric system and is released directly into the blood stream. This is where health problems begin because you are creating an imbalance.

Hemp seeds or Hemp Milk is readily available at your health food store or your supermarket. Buy hulled hemp seed. Making Hemp Milk for your self is fast and easy and can be done at a quarter of the cost of buying Hemp Milk. Natural sweeteners like maple syrup or honey can be added to taste and you can also flavour them with vanilla or almond extracts or cocoa powder for a supreme chocolate dream.

Ingredients

1 cup of hulled Hemp Hearts.
4 cups of water. pinch of sea salt.
1-2 tbs. of maple syrup or honey.
1 tsp. of vanilla or almond extract.

Procedure

Soak hemp hearts in 1 cup of water over night in the fridge. Blend ingredients and strain.
Straining is optional, the left over Hemp Hearts can be eaten or used as an ingredient for other recipes. There you have it, hemp milk ready for consumption. Check out my YouTube video on how to make it.

How to Make Hemp Milk

The Cannabis Burger

This is one of my favorite medibles because it completely masks the flavor of Marijuana. It is a joy to eat if you are a meat eater. It is absolutely delicious.

Use regular hamburger with about 20% fat content. Cannabinoids are fat-soluble so you need the fat content for the cannabinoids to bind too.

Ingredients

1lb. regular hamburger
1 egg.
½ cup of breadcrumbs
6-8 tsp. Canna flour
¾ tsp. sea salt
½ tsp. black pepper
½ tsp. crushed chilies
1 tbs. organic soya sauce
1 tsp. crushed garlic

Place the ingredients in a bowl and mix really, really well. This recipe will make four ¼ pound hamburgers.

Form meat into patties and cook on a barbeque, a grill, an open frying pan or a broiler. Start with a hot grill and sear the pattie to the grill. This will seal the hamburger. Because the hamburger contains breadcrumbs it will absorb the juice and the fat from the hamburger. Normally these juices will rise to the top of the hamburger but because of the absorption this will not happen.

The hamburger will take a few minutes on each side. Turn the hamburger once, searing the burger a second time. Cook the hamburgers until they are medium well to well done.

Do not cut the hamburger pattie open to check to see if it is done because most of the juice will run off. Just gently press down on the hamburger and if it bounces back like a cake it is done.

Toast a whole wheat Kaiser and top with your favorite dressings.

Serve with a salad, fries or potato chips.

Enjoy.

Check the link for an instructional video on how to make The Cannabis Burger.

Cannabis Burger

Cannabis Meatballs

If you don't like the taste of Marijuana then this is another recipe that you will enjoy.

Ingredients

1/2lb regular hamburger
1/2lb. ground pork
1 egg
½ cup bread crumbs.
¾ tsp. sea salt
½ tsp. black pepper
1 tsp. crushed chilies.
1 tbs. organic soya Sauce
1 tsp. chopped parsley.
1 tsp. fresh chopped basil
½ tsp. fresh chopped oregano
6-8 tsp. Canna flour

Place the ingredients in a bowl and mix well so you have an even distribution of your ingredients. Form small meatballs, the more service area the more taste. Broil them or cook them on a hot grill, searing, sealing and caramelizing with high heat for flavor, flavor.

Finish them of by simmering them in your favorite spaghetti sauce.

Serve with whole-wheat pasta or in a meatball sandwich.

Canna Flour

For making canna flour you can use leaf, sugar shake or bud or a combination of the two or three. I use a mix of sugar shake and bud.

I will dry the herb out completely in the oven. Dry it out below 175°F if you do not wish to decarboxylate the marijuana. Heat between 175°F and 200°F if you wish to decarboxylate the marijuana.

Place the herb in a high-speed blender and grind it up until it is a fine consistency. I then sift the canna flour thru a cake sifter and there you have it. Canna flour fit for consumption.

I have found that you can replace up to a third of the flour with canna flour in your recipes and it will work out fine from a technical perspective. So if you are making bread, cakes, cookies, muffins or what have you, the same rule applies.

I am developing a line of baked goods and I will be loading this book up with more recipes as I develop them so don't forget to turn on your automatic updates.

Marijuana and Spirituality

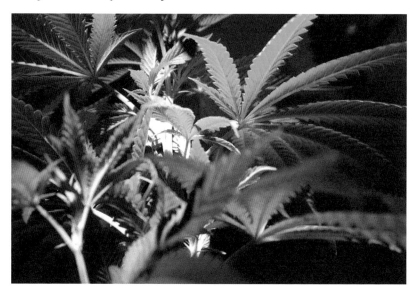

When I talk about spirituality I am not referring to peoples religious believe system. I am referring to the energy that flows thru our body that creates pure consciousness. What ever you are, Christian, Muslim, Hindu or Buddhist this energy flows thru us all, it is universal.

We are vibrational beings of pure consciousness, generating and working with energy to shape our world.

We are vibrational beings and marijuana plants are also vibrational beings that manifest's energy. Energy is basically a language like music is language. Marijuana resonates on a multitude of frequencies that is harmonious to our electromagnetic field. Marijuana opens our chakras. Chakras are like gateways in your body that open and close allowing energy to flow in and out.

After smoking marijuana our chakras can double in size, providing up to twice as much energy flowing thru out our body and provide us with energy to heal.

Spiritualists refer to the marijuana plant as a knowledge plant, a teacher plant and that is because the plants energy field contains electrical and chemical information that brings us into a calm, peaceful state of awareness.

Marijuana reduces resistance. Resistance creates tension, tension creates stress, stress creates pain and stress inhibits the flow of vital energy in our body.

Marijuana is a sedative that relaxes you, the tension is released and the pain melts away. A body at ease is free of dis-ease.

When the mind is calm and the body is relaxed the mind and body begins to heal. When the mind and body is relaxed it is open to the healing energy that abounds us.

There are many chakras located thru out the body, but what we should be primarily concerned about is the seven primary chakras. Each chakra channels energy to a different system in the body.

If a chakra is congested or depleted it will have a negative affect on the system it feeds energy too. Too much energy can be just as crippling as not enough energy and the objective is to always maintain a balance.

A healthy chakra system creates a strong energy field that will protect you from your environment. This energy flows outside of the physical body and is your body of light. We are beings of light and our physical body is a vibrational manifestation of that light. You are the light and you can expand several feet beyond the physical plane of existence.

Modern science can now measure this aura of light that we manifest. We can also take pictures of it. Energy healers know that disease shows up in the aura long before the disease manifests itself in the physical realm.

When your body of light becomes depleted you become vulnerable to disease. Using marijuana can be very effective at restoring balance and restoring the levels of energy in your body.

This energy is well known as Chi or Qi. Different cultures have different words for it. Science identifies it as subtle energy and they are just beginning to understand its true nature. Subtle energy can travel 400 light years in about a quarter of a second. Try wrapping your mind around that.

Starting at the base of the chakra system is the root chakra, which resonates into the colour red. The root chakra primarily channels energy into the eliminative system.

The second chakra is the sex chakra, which resonates into the colour orange. The sex chakra primarily channels energy into the reproductive system. It is here where life is created.

The third chakra is the solar plexus and resonates into the colour yellow and primarily channels energy into the digestive system.

The fourth chakra is the heart chakra and resonates into the colour green. The heart chakra primarily channels energy into circulation.

The fifth chakra is the throat chakra and resonates into the colour blue. The throat chakra primarily channels energy into respiration.

The sixth chakra is the third eye chakra and resonates into the colour indigo. The third eye chakra primarily channels energy into cognition, the endocrine system and the central and peripheral nervous system.

The seventh chakra is the crown chakra and resonates into the colour white. White is a reflection of all the colours in the spectrum and channels energy into the immune system. This light can also appear to be violet or purple. White light can also channel energy thru out the entire body and can be used to treat all the systems in the body.

Rising up or tuning in to a higher frequency or a higher level of consciousness only imposes a hierarchy, which in turn imposes a governing body of power that will control your behaviour. Expanding your knowledge, expanding your awareness, expanding consciousness is key to enlightenment. Growth expands in every direction just like those big fat juicy buds, bathing in full spectrum light.

I hope I have helped you gain a basic understanding of how energy works in the body and how marijuana can enhance the mind and bodies ability to make a recovery. I am a Qi Gong practitioner so working with energy is kind of my thing.

Herbal Enemas

An enema is a method used to flush waste out of the colon. The average person may have up to 10 pounds or more of non-eliminated waste in the large intestine. An enema cleans up the colon and induces bowel movements, leaving you feeling cleaner, lighter, and healthier almost immediately. The main job of the colon is to absorb water and nutrients from food and remove waste and toxins. Over the years, the colon walls can become encrusted with non-eliminated waste, making it sluggish and inefficient. When this happens you could experience allergies, depression, headaches, fatigue, nausea, loss of appetite, inability to concentrate, indigestion, irritability, stomach pains, swelling, weight problems. backache, bloating, constipation, candida yeast infections, flatulence, haemorrhoids, sinus congestion, skin conditions and unpleasant breath.

The ancient Egyptians believed that all diseases were caused by tainted, unwanted additions to food, or too much food, and understood how an enema could offer relief. Physicians prescribed enemas on a regular basis to treat serious illnesses.

Ancient regions in Africa, Greece, Babylonia, India, and China used enemas. American Indians performed enemas. Louis XIV used enemas in his lifetime and stayed healthy throughout. Even the vivacious Mae (Mary Jane) West started every day with a morning enema.
While the medical community has somehow disconnected itself from the benefits of enemas, administering enemas at home is save, effective and growing in popularity since it is a very healthy thing to do.

There are two types of enemas:

The **cleansing enema** is retained for a short period of time until your natural peristaltic movement eliminates both the water and the loose fecal material. It is used to gently flush out the colon.

The **retention enema** is held in the body for longer. For example, the famous "coffee enema" is retained for approximately 15 minutes or can also be left in and absorbed. Coffee enemas are an example of short-term (15 minute) retention enemas. Coffee enemas were made popular by Max Gerson, who used them with cancer patients to open the bile ducts and increase bile flow, helping to rid the liver of impurities.

Examples of *cleansing* enemas:

Apple Cider Vinegar in Water - Helps with viral conditions and to clear mucous from the body. Great if you suffer from nasal congestion or asthma.

Burdock Root - Helps to eliminate calcium deposits and purify blood.

Catnip Tea - Relieves constipation and congestion and will bring down a high fever.

Lemon Juice - Just what you need to clean the colon of fecal matter, balance its pH, and detoxify the system.

Examples of *retention* enemas:

Coffee - A coffee solution (we mean a good organic breakfast blend, not decaf or instant) stimulates both the liver and the gallbladder to release toxins (15 minutes only).

Minerals - This is one you will want to retain permanently. It helps rebuild the energy of the adrenals and the thyroid.

Probiotic - Perfect for candidiasis and other yeast infections.

Red Raspberry Leaf- High in iron, great for the eyes, and particularly helpful for women.

Fresh Raw Marijuana: A very efficient way to absorb the many medicinal compounds found in marijuana.

Each enema requires a slightly different method, but the results for each will be glorious. When a smaller amount of liquid is retained indefinitely, people in the biz call this an implant. One cup of liquid with a probiotic, minerals, or something green with chlorophyll (like wheat grass) or (fresh raw marijuana) makes an excellent implant. They'll quickly have you on your way to a happier, healthier colon.

Herbal enemas are for more than just cleansing the colon. Herbal enemas are a very efficient way to achieve healing effects because the active substances in the herbs are absorbed by the intestinal walls and are absorbed directly into the blood stream.

When herbs are taken orally, some of the active substances are altered, weakened, or destroyed by gastric juices before they can be absorbed into the system.

Once administered, hold the herbal enema for as long as you can. Ten to fifteen minutes. The longer you can hold it the better. This will allow for more absorption of the active ingredients.

If you have not done a recent colon cleanse or enema, it is recommended to do a cleansing enema before administering a herbal enema to achieve better effects. This way, you will clear out the majority of the fecal matter before administering the herbal enema and more of the herbal solution will be absorbed.

Use filtered de-chlorinated water for your cleansing enema.

Avoid using enemas during acute flare-ups of inflammatory bowel conditions. Most herbs are contraindicated during pregnancy and breastfeeding. If you are pregnant, consult a health-care practitioner before administering herbal enemas.

Herbs are potent and anal administration is very effective, so you have to know what you are doing. You should consult a herbalist before administering medicinal herbs.

How to Prepare a Marijuana Herbal Enema

If you are using a juicer, juice enough fresh raw marijuana to make one ounce of marijuana juice.

Mix the marijuana juice with eight ounces of filtered de-chlorinated water.

Administer the enema.

If you are using a high-speed blender, place up to eight leaves of fresh raw marijuana with eight ounces of water and a few ice cubes, pulsate until juiced. This method should be done quickly to prevent the marijuana from decarboxylating.

Administer the enema.

You may want to warm up the enema solution a little for comfort but beware, heat decarboxylates marijuana, it may have a narcotic effect and it may be very potent since the method of application is highly efficient. Don't worry too much, marijuana doesn't begin to decarboxylate until it reaches 175°F.

How To Prepare A Coffee Enema

Bring to a boil one quart of filtered non-chlorinated water. Add three heaping tablespoons of organic coffee. Boil for fives minutes and let it cool down to room temperature. Filter the coffee and administer, making sure the coffee is not too hot.
When administering enemas you can use an enema bottle, an enema bag or an enema bucket.

Fluid Amounts For Large-Volume Enemas

Infants: 50 - 150 ml.
Toddlers: 250 - 350 ml.
Children: 300 - 500 ml.
Adolescents: 500 - 750 ml.
Adults: 750 - 1,000 ml.

Suppositories

Excessive heat and the gastric system will destroy up to eighty percent of the cannabinoids found in marijuana. For this reason people will use a suppository, made from infused canna coconut oil would be best. It is as simple as sliding it up your butt, you may want to give yourself a cleansing enema first. Start out with a very low dosage because the cannabinoids will be absorbed directly into the bloodstream, making it at least four times more effective.

Marijuana and Addiction

So far, I have talked about the many benefits and the many ways you can use marijuana as a medicine and a source of food. Medical marijuana is saving peoples life's. No doubt about it, putting the political, legal and economic agenda aside, marijuana is improving the quality of life for many people.

With that said, I can't help but feel responsible for looking at the big picture. I must be un-biased and see both sides of the coin, so I asked myself, I said self, what are the pitfalls associated with using marijuana? Now I wasn't too highly motivated to go there but my thirst for knowledge is unquenchable.

Can marijuana be addictive? There are different levels of addiction. Marijuana isn't biologically addictive like heroin but you can develop a dependency on marijuana that starts out as pleasure seeking behaviour but end up as obsessive compulsive behaviour.

Marijuana can increase your levels of dopamine by ten fold, leaving you feeling very euphoric.

Your brain is a communications network and the front part of your brain is called the cerebral cortex, which receives information from your senses, processes them and sends chemical and electrical messages to other parts of the brain. From the cerebral cortex the information travels towards the brain stem where your Medulla is located.

The Medulla has many functions and one of them is to determine right from wrong based on survival needs. If you do something right you are rewarded with an electrical impulse and a chemical message that releases chemicals like dopamine in your limbic system. The electrical impulse reinforces the behaviour by motivating you to repeat the behaviour.

When you do not achieve or accomplish your goals or if your behaviour has bad consequences your behaviour is punished with chemicals like adrenaline to discourage your behaviour. It is all about survival and this is how the brain works. It is a punishment and reward system that motivates behaviour much like Pavlov's theory of conditioning.

If you use a stimulant like marijuana you are basically hijacking your Limbic system. After prolonged use, you loose the ability to enjoy life's simple pleasures, the motivation drops, depression sets in and you are now using to feel normal.

To avoid developing a marijuana dependency, practise moderation and it is a good idea to dry out once in awhile. Stop using for a while and allow your brain to get back to normal naturally. Smoking recreationally is one thing but when you start smoking marijuana everyday, it is going to have some negative consequences that you need to watch out for.

If you are a medical user then your dependency is justified. You need the medication to make a recovery. Medical marijuana is far less invasive then most pharmaceutical medications and medicinal marijuana can be more effective in most cases. You have to weigh the pros and cons and decide for yourself if medical marijuana will benefit you or diminish you.

When you are dying of cancer or you are in excruciating pain, medical marijuana can benefit you as a narcotic.

There are also many ways to medicate with medicinal marijuana without the psychoactive effects that leads to compulsive behaviour.

You can avoid decarboxylating your herb or you can consume medical marijuana in its fresh raw form, which is completely non-psychoactive and you still get the medicinal benefits, other then the euphoria. The feeling of being healthy and vibrant again feels better then a euphoric feeling that is blanketing an underlying condition.

Because marijuana is fat soluble it takes longer to withdraw but it is easy to manage compared to a tobacco, alcohol or a heroin addiction.

Marijuana consumed moderately is beneficial and is very effective at harm reduction when being used to come off harmful drugs like alcohol, opiates and amphetamines.

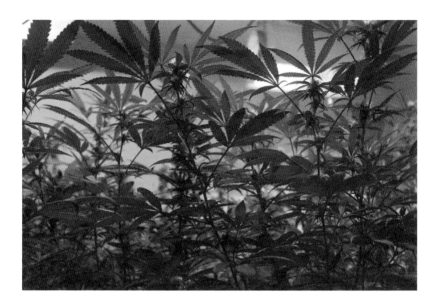

Summary

Marijuana can be a fairly heavy sedative but the dosage can easily be controlled. Society is at a fast pace and I don't think the government wants us chilling too hard. They would rather us just take the edge off with opiates.

Marijuana if consumed fresh and raw is non psychoactive and it will restore the imbalance that you are suffering from. Marijuana will feed your endocannabinoid system, which in turn will improve functionality.

It doesn't matter what you have been diagnosed with, marijuana will enable the mind and body to heal itself. Regenerate.

Fresh raw marijuana is the cure. Juice it or eat it in your salads.

I have taught you how to prepare medicinal marijuana in a safe and effective manner.

You have learned how to make extracts and infusions.

You have learned about the benefits of eating and juicing fresh raw marijuana and I have given you easy effective recipes to try for yourself.

With the preparations that you have learned how to make, you can fuse your medicine into just about anything like beverages, cakes, muffins, cookies and even savory dishes.

Remember, if you cook at high temperatures your medicine will not be as effective.

I am currently creating recipes that provide a vital source of nutrition.

If you smoke or vaporize your marijuana it will not be as effective as a medicine. Smoking marijuana is therapeutic and has many health benefits but it is not going to cure chronic illnesses.

Ingesting medicinal marijuana is more effective as a medicine and is safe with no harmful side effects.

I believe in the power of holistic medicine and I believe that everyone should have access to natural remedies. Nutrition is the new medical model, the new science, based on regeneration of the human body. Every species on earth has the ability to regenerate. Why do we need doctors for that?

I understand that corporations and their political representatives have made this vital plant un-accessible for most people. These are people who are dying or suffering from serious illnesses, or they are trying to help loved ones, like their parents, or their children recover from crippling diseases with fatal consequences.

It is a serious problem that needs to be addressed and the only solution is to de-schedule marijuana. Marijuana is a herb, a vegetable that is a complete food source. It should be classified and regulated as food under the food and drug administration act.

If people want to use marijuana as a narcotic they have to change the plants chemistry by applying heat. Marijuana does not become a narcotic until it has been decarboxylated, only then can it be classified as a controlled substance we know as cannabis. A narcotic with over 5,000 patents registered so far. The plant itself cannot be patented, but what the plant can be used for, can be patented.

I have smoked over a million dollars worth of weed in my time. I grew most of it myself, otherwise I wouldn't of been able to afford it. I suggest you grow your own medicine. It becomes affordable and you have full control over the quality. Be sure to check out my grow book. The Medical Marijuana Growers Guide. From seed to harvest.

Peace And Prosperity For All.

Bibliography

Chef Derek Butt. http://www.chefderekbutt.com

http://www.youtube.com/user/masterchefb1

Dr. Courteny. http://www.cannabisinternational.org/index.php

Dr. McAllister. http://www.cpmc.org/professionals/research/programs/science/sean.html

Dr. Hergenrather. http://medicalmarijuana.com/medical-marijuana-directory/listingDetails.cfm?lisID=739

Dr. Melamede. http://www.uccs.edu/~rmelamed/

Dr. Guzman. http://www.immugen.com/blog-for-cannabinoids-research/tags/Dr.-Manuel-Guzman/

Dr. Abrams. http://www.ucsfhealth.org/donald.abrams

Dr. Bearman. http://www.davidbearmanmd.com/publications.htm

Dr. Nagarkatti. http://pmi.med.sc.edu/PNagarkatti.asp

Dr. Mckuriya. http://mikuriyamedical.com/about/can_write.html

Pubmed http://www.ncbi.nlm.nih.gov/pubmed

Net Work

Check out my YouTube channel for instructional videos on everything covered in this book and then some. Also available to you are tips and tricks for cultivating medicinal marijuana. My videos are informative and entertaining.

I am also a composer, a musician and a producer. I wrote the music in my videos. I studied music therapy at Capilano University and I think you will find my music, like most music to be therapeutic. May be not. I was kind of angry when I wrote it. It was therapeutic for me.

Now that I am well medicated, I am looking forward to writing my next album.

http://derekbutt.com

YouTube Playlists:

Extracts and Infusions

Cannabis Infused Cuisine

Fresh Raw Marijuana

Medical Marijuana Growing Tips

Facebook, **YouTube**, **Twitter**, **Linkedin**　　**Google+**,　**chefderekbutt.com** **themedicalmarijuanaguide.com**

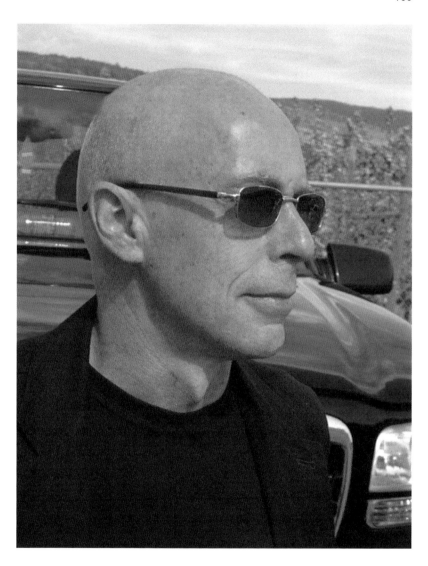

Chef Derek Butt.

The End

Made in the USA
Columbia, SC
08 September 2017